NO MORE KIDNEY STONES

John S. Rodman, M.D.
and
Cynthia Seidman, M.S., R.D.
with
Rory Jones

John Wiley & Sons, Inc.

New York • Chichester • Brisbane • Toronto • Singapore

Library of Congress Cataloging-in-Publication Data:

Rodman, John S.
    No more kidney stones / by John S. Rodman and Cynthia Seidman with Rory Jones.
        p.   cm.
    Includes bibliographical references.
    ISBN 0-471-12587-3 (pbk. : alk. paper)
    1. Kidneys—Calculi—Prevention.   I. Seidman, Cynthia.
II. Jones, Rory.   III. Title.
RC916.R63   1996
616.6'2205—dc20   95-52786

CONTENTS

PART TWO

THE PLAN

PART THREE

MEDICINES, SPECIALISTS, AND PROCEDURES

PREFACE

When I started practicing nephrology twenty years ago, kidney stones that did not pass often required open surgery. Dietary advice usually consisted of "drink more water and eliminate all of the dairy products from your diet." Most of the people I treated for multiple stone episodes were given drugs to reduce their urinary calcium.

Today, most surgery has been replaced by shock wave or laser fragmentation of stones, and we know that reducing calcium is unnecessary for many people and may actually aggravate the problem for a few stone formers. When a prescription is written, it is more likely to be for a naturally occurring substance than for a drug.

As I treated more patients with recurring stone disease, I realized that at least 75 percent of my patients stopped making stones with dietary advice alone. It became apparent that the key to helping people to avoid kidney stones was not going to be the prescription I wrote on a medical pad but the finding of an *acceptable* way for them to change the way they ate—and in some cases the way they lived. I emphasize the word *acceptable* because many "ideal" diets represent such a departure from most people's food habits that they are totally impracticable.

No other disease has a more critical relation to diet. The frequency of stone disease has increased in parallel with the richer Western diet. It is a rare emergency room in an industrialized nation that does not see several patients with colicky pain from kidney stones every week.

As I mapped out diet and fluid recommendations for my patients, many of them wanted something they could refer to when they had questions. They wanted more explanation for oxalate tables, protein control, and fluid guidelines. They asked what they could order in Italian, French, and Chinese restaurants. Family members requested cooking information. The short summary I gave to patients— "Dietary Guidelines for the Stone Former"—became the first notes for this book.

I started to look for patients that might characterize the eating habits of various stone formers, such as the forty-year-old man who began making stones when his weight increased or the middle-aged woman who drank 2 quarts of iced tea a day. I also saw certain lifestyle patterns that led to the formation of kidney stones. Most sufferers fit one of these patterns. If you can find yourself in this book and make the appropriate changes, you will probably markedly decrease your chance of making stones.

The second reason for writing this book was to find ways for people to stay on the wagon. One of the more difficult aspects of preventing stone disease is keeping people motivated. Frequently, people will follow guidelines religiously for the first three or four months after a stone episode and, when the memory of that awful pain begins to fade, return to the same habits that got them into trouble.

However, I have found that the people who are most successful in eliminating stone episodes from their lives are the ones who understand how and why stones form in the first place. I have therefore tried to explain the "science" in a simple manner that can be used for reference. I was a chemistry major in college, which is one reason why I chose the subspecialty of nephrology, the body's chemistry, after my training in internal medicine. I hope this book will enable you to understand why your urine makes crystals and how these crystals grow big enough to become kidney stones.

I am grateful to my patients who have taught me to make my explanations simple enough for the nonscientist to grasp easily. They have also pointed out where my recommendations for diet and lifestyle changes were too ideal or impractical. In turn, I have often had to convince some of them that certain "impractical" changes were necessary if they were to prevent more procedures and more trips to the emergency room. It is from this give-and-take with thousands of patients that the suggestions in this book have evolved.

Nevertheless, there is no substitute for advice from a physician who knows your individual case. You may also need to coordinate a stone prevention program with other aspects of your health. For example, if you have diabetes, your diet will have to be appropriate to that problem as well. Therefore, if you have any questions, you should discuss the information in this book with your own physician. Your doctor can help determine which dietary emphasis is most appropriate for your own care.

ACKNOWLEDGMENTS

There are many physicians who have taught me what I know about stone disease and assisted me in my clinical research. I wish I could thank all of them. Some deserve special mention:

Dr. Charles Y. C. Pak, director of the Section of Mineral Metabolism of the University of Texas School of Medicine, whose laboratory has performed the analyses for several of the clinical studies I have published in the book. He has been a good friend and mentor.

Dr. Marcus Reidenberg, chief of the Division of Clinical Pharmacology, and Dr. E. Daracott Vaughan, Jr., director of the Division of Urology at Cornell University School of Medicine, both of whom have encouraged and enabled the research.

My collaborators on this book, Cynthia Seidman and Rory Jones, and I would also like to thank others who have contributed their time, patience, and expertise to our effort:

PJ Dempsey, our editor, who has supported this book and guided its progress.

Faith Hamlin, who believed in the concept from the start.

Richard LaRocco, who works in the medical art and photography department of New York Hospital/Cornell Medical Center and did the illustrations.

My collaborators and I would also like to thank our families for their patience and help over the past year, including Irwin Iroff, David Jones, and, in particular, Sylvia Rodman. She was the first subject in our pilot study of the safety of calcium supplementation for osteoporosis in women who had previously made stones. Her support, encouragement, and good-humored willingness to try new diets were instrumental in the development and completion of this book.

Finally, we would like to thank the many patients who volunteered to be interviewed so that we could translate their problems, eating patterns, and experiences into the case examples in this book.

ABOUT THIS BOOK

The words in *italics* throughout the text are common technical terms that you may encounter. They are listed in the Glossary for easy reference.

The metric system has been used as the standard for measurement throughout the text. A conversion table is provided in Appendix A.

Throughout the text we emphasize the need to consult with your physician for a proper diagnosis and treatment of kidney stones. This is an extra reminder that no medication, procedure, diet, or supplement should be taken or undertaken without consulting a doctor or other qualified professional.

Many people with kidney stones were interviewed for this book. Their names and other details have been changed to protect their privacy.

PART ONE

WHAT YOU NEED TO KNOW ABOUT KIDNEY STONES

May I govern my passions with absolute sway,
And grow wiser and better, as strength wears away,
Without gout or stone, by a gentle decay.
—WALTER POPE (C. 1630–1714)

1

THE KIDNEY STONE BOOM

I drink gallons of milk a day. I love cheese, especially
Brie. I love cheeseburgers. I often go out for a big lunch
and grab a yogurt for dinner. I like raspberry jam on
toast and I love peanuts. I've always sort of pooh-poohed
dietary counseling. Listen, I smoke a pack and a half of
cigarettes a day: telling me not to put raspberry jam on
my toast is sort of ridiculous to my way of thinking.
But the pain was the type I couldn't stand. I couldn't sit
and I couldn't lie down. It came in waves. If I'm good,
maybe I won't get these damn things again.

*—*Sara, 28

You get different advice from different doctors. It's
confusing. About four years after my first episode, I saw a
urologist in the country who did an X ray and found three
more stones in my kidney. He wanted to do lithotripsy to
break up the stones. But, when I got back to the city and
saw my regular doctor, he felt the three stones were too
small to zap. The doctor in the country wanted to zap
them, the doctor in the city felt they were too small. I was
kind of caught between a stone and a hard place. . . .
   What will really cut down my chance of getting stones
again?

*—*Peter, 44

It happened right in the middle of my summer holiday.
Just like the first episode. We weren't allowed to take stuff

3

on the beach to drink, so I'd sit down there sweating. I'd drink gallons of iced tea, though, whenever we weren't on the beach. Anyway, I was fine one minute, and the next minute I had this horrible pain and I was vomiting and had diarrhea. It came and it went, and came and went. But then it got worse and worse until I was on the floor.

I'm terrified of doctors. I'm terrified of hospitals. I don't want to know about it. I don't like the idea that I could be anywhere and go off like a time bomb like I did last summer. What do I do to never get another kidney stone?

—ANITA, 52

I'm an ex-college football player and all that stuff. Went into sales, great expense account, best restaurants, steaks—I was going for the world cholesterol record when it all stopped. The doctors said, if you can get your weight under control, you are going to be fine. I lost 35 pounds and thought that would do it. I put a little bit of it back on this year and then unfortunately this happened. I knew what it was—unless my wife and kids were sticking me in the back with a knife.

I'm going to take whatever precautions I need to take to avoid it again.

—CHRIS, 45

The torment of a kidney stone attack is not easily forgotten. It is often impossible to believe that something so little can cause so much pain. Most people who have suffered through such an episode are highly motivated to do anything necessary to avoid another attack. Unfortunately, despite their initial good intentions, people who have made a kidney stone are likely to make another.

A health problem since ancient times, kidney stones have afflicted many famous historical figures, including Benjamin Franklin, Isaac Newton, Peter the Great, and Louis XIV. X rays of Egyptian mummies dating back eight to ten thousand years ago show evidence of stones. "Cutting for the stone" is one of the oldest surgical procedures. Interestingly, the specialty of urology is the only one noted in the Hippocratic oath.

What Are Kidney Stones?

In the simplest of terms, kidney stones are composed of waste products—things the body does not need. Your kidneys normally eliminate these wastes in urine. When there is too much waste, or not enough fluid to flush it out, it comes together to form a "stone." Some of these stones are so small they are like grains of sand, or gravel. When the kidneys eliminate these stones, the pain can be excruciating. It is often compared, unfavorably, to childbirth or surgery without anesthesia.

Why Do Some People Get Kidney Stones?

Medical science cannot say with certainty why some people are prone to kidney stones. We do know that they tend to run in families, indicating a genetic predisposition to the condition. There is also a link to chronic dehydration and certain types of eating disorders.

Today, approximately one in fifteen people in the industrialized world will develop kidney stones. In some communities, that number is one in five. More than a million Americans are hospitalized each year for treatment of the condition. And, what was once predominantly a male disease is now crossing the sexual barrier.

Why are we seeing such a growth in kidney stone disease?

The Stone "Boom"

Since World War II, the incidence of stone disease has been increasing dramatically in the Western industrialized nations. In a country like Germany, an adult male has a one in ten chance of making a kidney stone in his lifetime. This is a country that saw very little stone disease before the 1950s. A number of studies have been done and they have clearly connected this increase to what people are eating.

As we eat richer diets, we must deal with more wastes. And wastes come through our kidneys and out in our urine. While this is an oversimplification of the issues we discuss in this book, it focuses the main problem for most stone formers. The stone "boom" is tied to our diets.

In addition, while the medical treatment of existing stones is now extremely sophisticated, it is not the long-term answer to the problem of recurring stone disease. Lithotripsy, surgery, medication, and/ or painkillers can solve your immediate problem and alleviate your pain until the next episode occurs. After numerous episodes of renal colic (kidney stones), especially if the stones become infected, you can do permanent damage to one or both of your kidneys.

Prevention Is the Cure

You cannot cure a predisposition to kidney stones. We cannot change the fact that some people are prone to stone disease because of genetics or an underlying medical condition. In some cases an anatomic abnormality can be surgically corrected, but this is not the cause of the majority of kidney stones. You *can* change your diet and actually prevent a stone recurrence.

The Dietary Prescription

After many years of trying to find a medicine that would "cure" people of kidney stones, doctors found that two-thirds of patients seen with recurring stones stopped making them with basic dietary advice. The Mayo Clinic labeled this phenomenon the "stone clinic effect."

My experience is even better than the two-thirds figure. If people understand what causes stones and make the basic diet and lifestyle changes that we are recommending, they can prevent the recurrence of kidney stones. Only a handful need to take medication. While there are certain medical conditions that predispose some people to stone formation and make their special cases more difficult to control, even the toughest stone problems can be ameliorated with the advice in this book.

Preventing Kidney Stones

Preventing kidney stones requires an understanding of the problem and the specific changes that you will have to make to avoid a recurrence.

Step One

I have found that people who understand how and why they made kidney stones are more successful in preventing a recurrence. They are able to determine how aggressively their dietary and lifestyle habits must be changed. Therefore, the first part of this book explains what kidney stones are, how and why they form, what habits and behaviors raise the risk of attack, and the dietary and lifestyle elements that promote stone formation. We then help you assess whether you are at low or high risk of another attack.

Step Two

The next step consists in targeting the specific dietary and lifestyle changes that will prevent your type of stone disease. The Master Plan for kidney stone prevention, outlined in Part Two, is a dietary prescription that has evolved and been refined over twenty years of clinical practice.

Any diet is, by definition, an inhibition of spontaneous behavior. You cannot eat *what* you want *when* you want it. I was explaining certain foods that might trigger another episode to one patient who told me, "I'm the type of person that if you told me right now I could never have rhubarb again I'd suddenly want rhubarb. I hate rhubarb."

Certain desserts, large portions, second helpings, cheating on weekends, and certain forbidden foods all play a part. You must be motivated and willing to change certain eating and lifestyle habits.

Commitment to Change

Because many people are given medicines or must undergo procedures to get rid of stones, Part Three of this book explains the medical specialties, medicines, and procedures that you may encounter.

If you are reading this book, you have either made or passed a kidney stone or want to help someone who has had kidney stones. That process is usually sufficient motivation. We are asking you to make a commitment to change certain eating and lifestyle habits that contribute to stone formation. Most of you will find the necessary changes quite easy to accomplish. The Master Plan is easy to follow and fits into the way people actually live and work.

I have found that the resolve of many people often recedes along with the memory of their pain. For this reason, I recommend keeping this book in a convenient spot and rereading not only the dietary advice but the case histories. They may serve to remind you of the discomfort—and extreme pain—that you are missing.

2

THE URINARY SYSTEM

I never thought about my kidneys before.
You take them for granted until something happens.

The urinary system cleans the body of wastes. It gets rid of every-thing that the body does not need, in order to maintain balance in the rest of the systems. For instance, your body does not need 16 ounces of meat at dinner. The waste products of that meat will be circulated to your kidneys to be eliminated. And some of these waste products are the building blocks of kidney stones.

The Urinary System and How It Works

If we are to understand what goes wrong in the urinary system to cause kidney stones, it is important to see how this hardworking system normally operates to keep the body healthy.

The Kidneys

The kidneys are the main organ of the urinary system. We are born with two kidneys that lie against the back of the abdominal wall, just above the waist. Each kidney is about the size of a small grapefruit.

Your kidneys do not make urine—they make clean blood. This often comes as a surprise to people. Yet this concept is critical to the management of kidney stones.

If you see smoke coming out of a power plant, you know that it is working. The plant does not manufacture smoke, it is simply a by-product of its workings. Similarly, if we see urine, we know that the

9

kidney is working. But urine is a by-product of the workings of the kidney, not its main industry.

The kidneys have two basic functions:

1. Cleaning out toxic substances from the blood
2. Keeping the things your body *does* need in proper balance

For example, if you eat something that could be poisonous to your system, like lead, the kidney's job is to get rid of it and not let it accumulate in your body. Substances that the body needs constantly, such as sodium, must be kept at healthy levels. (See Chapter 3 for more on balance.)

How the Kidneys Work

Your blood transports nutrients and oxygen to the cells of the body and carries away waste material that the body does not need. These waste materials are then brought back to the kidney to be excreted.

Under normal resting conditions, about 25 percent, or one-fourth, of your blood flows into the kidneys through the *renal arteries*. The kidneys filter the blood flow from your heart through a sophisticated system that removes unneeded waste products from the blood and returns clean blood to the body via the *renal veins*. In the process, it discards what is not needed as urine via the *ureter*. (See Figure 1.)

Filtration

The kidneys work by filtering the blood that comes into each kidney through a very efficient system of microscopic *nephrons*.

Each kidney has about one million nephrons, which are the workhorses of the kidney. The nephrons eventually join together and lead into the collecting ducts that finally empty into the *renal* or *kidney pelvis*. By the time the fluid in the nephrons has passed through the collecting ducts to reach the kidney pelvis, it has become urine.

Urine

Urine is composed of water, salt, small amounts of acid, and a variety of waste products like urea, oxalate, uric acid, potassium, magnesium, creatinine, and other unwanted things (e.g., lead).

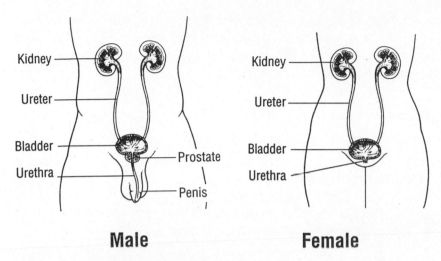

Male   **Female**

Figure 1.   The Male and Female Urinary Tracts
Both the male and female urinary tracts consist of two kidneys, which drain
through their respective ureters into a bladder that is a holding sack. The
difference between the male and female urinary tracts lies in the outflow from
the bladder through the urethra. The female urethra is a short structure that
drains easily to the outside world. The male urethra is much more complicated, as it must pass through the prostate gland and then through the penis
before reaching the external orifice.

The composition and amount of urine changes as the kidneys
compensate for changes in what you eat and drink, as well as lifestyle
changes and illness. (See the section "How the Kidneys Keep the
Body in Balance" in Chapter 3.) Urine accumulates in the collecting
system of the kidney, which includes the pelvis and *calyces*. The
kidney pelvis has smooth muscle that periodically contracts and
squeezes urine into the ureter. Additional muscular contractions of
the ureter propel the urine into the bladder.

The Bladder

The *bladder* is where urine is stored until it is excreted. It is a tem-
porary storage space that tells you when it is full. The *detrussor muscle*
makes the bladder contract and expel urine. (See "Prostatitis" in
Chapter 11.)

Stones rarely become trapped in the female bladder because the
outflow of the female bladder is quite simple. The outflow of the

male bladder is more complicated because it involves the prostate gland and the penis. (See Chapter 11, "Men and Stones.") When there is an obstruction of urine, there is the potential for stones to become stuck in the male ureter and bladder.

Reflux

Urine in the bladder should never go back "upstream," which is called *reflux*. There is a triangular muscle structure called a *trigone* that seals the ureters when you urinate and stops urine from reentering the kidneys. Some people, however, have a congenital defect in the trigone that allows reflux; this condition may predispose those people to kidney stones as well as kidney infections.

The Balance Concept

The kidneys preserve a very delicate balance in the body. They compensate for your food and fluid intake in order to maintain this balance.

For instance, if you drink a great deal of water, there is a greater volume of urine. If you eat a lot of salt (that bag of potato chips that disappeared during the football game), more comes out in the urine. If you eat a lot of protein, more of the waste products of protein metabolism come out in your urine. The body must stay in zero balance, or you would blow up with water or become ill from an excess of salt.

The only time you don't have zero balance is when the body is sick. For instance, if you get food poisoning, the body becomes dehydrated and loses salt and other minerals necessary for balance and good health. Patients with chronic bowel disease lose fluid and minerals through diarrhea.

Fluids and Balance

When the body is deprived of water, the kidneys conserve fluid and make a more concentrated urine (one that contains little fluid). A concentrated urine is dangerous for the stone former, as kidney stones are much more likely to form there than in a dilute urine. (See Chapter 5, "How and Why Kidney Stones Form.")

We often assume that the amount of water you take in is equal to the amount of urine. This is true if someone is not active: The fluid in equals the fluid out. At rest, the amount of water generated from the metabolism of food and drink is roughly equal to the amount you lose in stool and perspiration.

That assumption falls apart if you work in a hot office or factory, are near a hot oven, are on the beach, or for any other reason are perspiring heavily. Then you are losing a lot of water through your skin. If you are exercising strenuously, the kidneys will return more fluid to the body to enable it to cool the surface of the skin through the sweat glands. The kidney compensates by reducing the urinary volume. You may notice that you urinate less when you are sweating heavily. In these situations, the amount of fluid you are taking in does *not* equal the amount of urine you make. The kidneys are balancing the amount of water, as well as sodium and other substances such as potassium, that the body needs for its activity level.

How Trouble Starts

The urinary tract is really the body's sewer system, and the kidney is the processing plant for waste disposal. The more waste the kidney must get rid of, and the less fluid volume it has to flush the waste out, the greater the chance that it will clog up.

I look at kidney stones as clogs in the urinary system. It is my goal to show you how to keep your sewer pipes unclogged.

3

HOW YOUR KIDNEYS BALANCE YOUR BODY

These urinary deposits indicate a general derangement of the system . . .
—*THE PEOPLE'S COMMON SENSE MEDICAL ADVISOR IN PLAIN ENGLISH*, R. V. PIERCE, M.D. (1895)

Your kidneys get rid of things that do not belong in your body and keep those that do in the proper proportions. This concept of balance is very important for the stone former to understand.

Try to imagine what would happen if your body were not kept at a constant composition. Let's say that you drank an extra quart of water each day and your kidneys did not increase the amount of water you eliminated to keep pace. Within a week, you would have gained 15 pounds and would be quite swollen. This is exactly what can happen with acute failure of the kidneys. Or, suppose you added just 1 tablespoon of table salt to your food each day, and the kidneys did not increase sodium excretion. Within a week, your blood would be as brackish as seawater and your brain would shrivel up, just as your skin does when you swim in the ocean.

It is important for you to remember that your kidneys play the main role in balancing your body chemistry. Without functioning kidneys, your body would be unable to rid itself of toxic substances, excess fluid, or excessive amounts of minerals such as salt. In many cases, this could become life threatening.

Why Balance Is Important

The machinery of the cell cannot work unless the blood's chemistry is constant. The pumps in cell membranes will not work. The mechanism that makes muscles contract will not work.

The body must stay in zero balance, and the kidneys are the main regulatory organs to accomplish that task.

Elements of Balance

The *digestive system* resembles a hollow tube that is open at both ends. The food and liquids we consume enter this tube via the mouth and are swallowed into the stomach, where they are broken down and sent to the intestines.

The intestine is a passageway for food where nutrients are absorbed. In the small and large intestine food and liquids are digested and absorbed by the body into the bloodstream and thereby circulated to the cells of the body. The nonabsorbed waste products of digestion accumulate in the large intestine and are prepared for excretion. They are excreted through the rectum/anus via the stool.

As we explained in Chapter 1, the waste products of cell metabolism are sent to the kidneys via the bloodstream and excreted in the urine.

The skin plays a role in the water balance of the body. It uses water as perspiration to cool the body and regulate its temperature. On a hot summer day or during vigorous exercise, you can sweat off several liters of water.

How the Kidneys Keep the Body in Balance

The ultimate control of balance in the body lies with the kidneys. If you are at home watching television and drink a quart of water, you will urinate approximately a quart of liquid. On the other hand, if you are out playing tennis and drink the same quart of water, you may lose half the water in perspiration. Your kidneys will guard the water balance of the body by producing only a pint of urine. This urine, though, will be much more concentrated; that is, the same amount of waste products will be eliminated in a smaller amount of fluid.

Urine equals what is eaten minus stool, perspiration and, rarely, other losses. (See Figure 2.)

The only time the body goes out of balance is when an illness such as *chronic diarrhea* or food poisoning strikes. Large amounts of fluid are then lost through the stool or vomiting. People who have had their colons removed and are left with an *ileostomy* also have a system that is out of balance because the colon, which is one of the chief places you absorb water, is bypassed. (See "Bowel Disease" in Chapter 9.) This extreme loss of fluids is often more than the kidneys can handle, and the body becomes out of balance because it is dehydrated. Dehydration is a common cause of stone formation.

The kidneys further guard the balance of the body by regulating the amounts of waste products of metabolism that are eliminated. Common waste products that are presented to the kidneys every day include urea, *creatinine*, uric acid, and oxalate. Other minerals presented to the kidneys include potassium, magnesium, sodium, and calcium. A number of these minerals will sound familiar to anyone who has had a kidney stone analyzed.

Calcium and Sodium

Calcium and sodium are each handled differently by the body. The amount of sodium (salt) that you eat equals the amount of sodium found in the urine, with a small amount lost through perspiration. Most of the salt you eat is absorbed by the intestines and eliminated in your urine, not your stool.

Unlike sodium, only a small fraction of the calcium you eat is absorbed by the body. Most is excreted via the intestines and stool. Therefore, the amount of calcium found in the urine is much less than the calcium you consume.

Calcium Absorption and Stone Formers

Some stone formers absorb a greater percentage of the calcium they eat than non–stone formers do. This calcium must then come out in

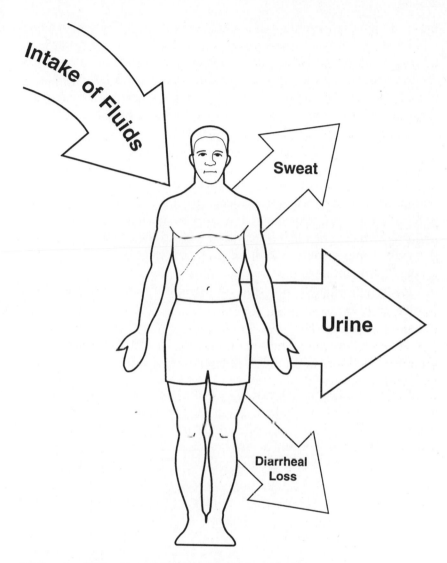

Figure 2.   What Goes In Equals What Comes Out
The amount of fluids you drink equals the amount of fluids leaving your body
through perspiration, diarrheal losses, and urine. Therefore, anything that
increases perspiration or diarrheal losses will reduce the amount of urine
coming out.

the urine. This situation is particularly true of young men who begin making stones in their twenties and early thirties. The body stays in balance because the kidney compensates by increasing calcium excretion. But the extra calcium in the urine increases the propensity to make stones. These people suffer from *absorptive hypercalciuria*. They are the one group of stone formers who need to be careful about the amount of dairy products they consume.

Acid and Base (pH)

Another balancing act that the kidneys perform is the relation of acid to base in the body. This balance is important to the body because it controls various chemical processes, such as the unloading of oxygen from hemoglobin in the blood so that it can reach the cells. It is especially important to the stone former because an acid urine affects the formation of both uric acid and calcium oxalate stones. (See Chapter 4.)

Common acidic substances are lemon juice and vinegar. A common basic substance is baking soda. Most foods break down into an acidic or an alkaline (base) residue. This is measured by your urinary pH.

The pH of water is 7.0, which is neutral. A pH below 7.0 is acidic, and a pH above 7.0 is alkaline, or basic. If you put an acid and a base together, they neutralize each other and form water. Conversely, water can be split into an acid and a base by certain chemical reactions such as those that occur in the stomach.

If you eat a diet high in animal protein, there is a large load of acid that must be excreted by the kidneys. We say that a carnivorous diet leaves an acid ash and a vegetarian diet leaves a basic ash. (The end product of metabolism is called an ash.) If you ate nothing but string beans, you would actually have a small load of base to excrete.

Normal urinary pH levels range between 5.0 and a little over 8.0. This varies with the time of day, food consumption, age, and other factors. When there is so much acid to excrete that the kidney cannot quite catch up, the urine is persistently acid. This is the case with some uric acid stone formers. (See "Uric Acid Stones" in Chapter 4.)

What Happens When the Body Gets Out of Balance

If the amount of fluid going into the body does not equal the net going out, the body is not in balance. The kidney must compensate for losses of fluids through the skin or bowel by making a small volume of urine. And this concentrated urine is what leads the kidney to make stones.

How to Keep Your Sewer System Unclogged

If you want to stop stone formation, there are two important things you must do:

- *Drink fluids.* You must take in enough fluid to compensate for all other losses and have enough left to make a dilute urine. This is the single most important piece of advice in this book.
- *Eliminate excess and unwanted "trash."* By altering what you "throw away" each day, you will alter the composition of your urine. If you eat more than you need, things will back up like a clogged drain and you will likely need a plumber. In medicine, the plumber is the urologist. Eating too much of certain foods is like putting coffee grounds and hair in your drain.

Our goal is to ensure that the things you eat and drink depart from your body without leaving any unwanted deposits behind in the urinary tract.

4

NOT ALL KIDNEY STONES ARE CREATED EQUAL

I've had three experiences with kidney stones. The first one was a uric acid stone. The second stone no one knows. The third one was a calcium oxalate stone. Actually, the next one I believe is going to be a rhinestone. And that is something I would not like you mentioning because I don't want people following me around with a strainer waiting for me to pee rhinestones. . . .

Kidney stones are composed of different substances and vary from one person to another. They can be as small as a grain of sand or bigger than a Ping-Pong ball. They range in color from yellow to reddish brown. Some are smooth, others have "horns." The medical name for kidney stones is *calculi,* which comes from the Latin word for stone or pebble.

Four Types of Kidney Stones

Kidney stones come in different varieties: (1) calcium-containing stones, (2) uric acid stones, (3) struvite, or infected, stones, and (4) cystine stones.

Seventy-five percent of the kidney stones that reach the stone analysis laboratory contain calcium oxalate as the predominant mineral. About 10 percent are composed of uric acid, and another 10 percent are struvite, or infected, stones. Often, a stone will contain a combination of these elements.

20

Cystine stones result from an uncommon hereditary metabolic disorder and account for fewer than 1 percent of stone cases. At least twenty different substances have been reported in kidney stones. Many are the results of rare diseases and beyond the scope of this book.

The stones in each of these categories have their own mineral composition, causes, and treatment approaches.

Calcium-Containing Stones

Most people have an intuitive understanding of what calcium is. It is found in milk, bones, oyster shells, and limestone. Most calcium stones are formed when the calcium combines with oxalate. Occasionally, calcium may also combine with *carbonate* or *phosphate*, substances that are found in the body naturally.

Hydroxyapatite and Carbonate Apatite Stones

Some calcium-containing stones contain a mineral called *apatite,* which is the same form of calcium that makes up your bones. The apatite crystal is what gives bone its strength.

Apatite is found in two different forms in kidney stones: *hydroxyapatite* and *carbonate apatite*. The presence of a small amount of these types of calcium is quite important, since it alerts your physician that you may have an unusual stone-forming process.

Apatite is found in five clinical situations:

1. With *renal tubular acidosis*, an inherited defect in the way the kidney handles acid
2. When there is an acquired problem from certain medications used to treat eye disease such as glaucoma
3. With *hyperparathyroidism*, a disorder of the calcium-controlling glands in your neck
4. With excessive use of antacids
5. When there are struvite (infected) stones caused by certain bacteria

Each of these medical conditions is discussed more fully in Chapter 9.

Most people with calcium stones will need to understand calcium oxalate and not these other unusual minerals.

Oxalate

Oxalate is a waste product of metabolism (see Chapter 8). It would be of no interest to us at all if it did not combine with the calcium you eat to make the crystals that form the most common type of kidney stone.

There are four sources of the oxalate that appears in the urine:

1. Large amounts of protein
2. Excess amounts of vitamin C
3. Waste products of general metabolism
4. Certain foods such as spinach, rhubarb, various berries, tea, cocoa, cola drinks, nuts, and others (See Chapters 8 and 17 and the Appendix, Table 2.)

A number of medical conditions may affect oxalate metabolism and the relative importance of each of these four sources of urinary oxalate. The most important is *bowel disease*, which leads to the overabsorption of dietary oxalate (see Chapter 9). Another is the rare genetic disorder called *primary hyperoxaluria,* or *oxalosis,* found mainly in children, where too much oxalate is generated. The kidneys of these children fill with stones, and they end up on *dialysis* at an early age. Some adults have high oxalate excretions (although not as high as the children with oxalosis) without any apparent explanation of it. They appear to have inherited an incomplete form of oxalosis.

When an excess amount of calcium and oxalate accumulates in the urine—whether through diet or physical disorders—it can form calcium oxalate crystals, which can grow into kidney stones. (See Chapter 5, "How and Why Stones Form.")

Uric Acid Stones

Uric acid is a product of metabolism. It results from the metabolism of the *purines,* which are found in all animal protein and many seeds and plants. Therefore, all meat breaks down into uric acid. The plant sources of uric acid are seeds such as beans, peas, and lentils.

Three factors favor uric acid stones:

1. The presence of a large amount of urate (uric acid) in the urine.

The consumption of large amounts of animal protein increases the amount of urate and results in a persistently acid urine.
2. A low urine volume, which makes the urine concentrated.
3. A continually acid urine. In a normal, healthy person, the urinary pH will rise to over 7.0 after a meal (referred to as the "postprandial alkaline tide"). Uric acid stone formers lose this rise, and their urinary pH remains at or close to 5.0 all of the time. (A pH below 7.0 is acidic.)

A number of medical conditions can lead to uric acid stones:

• *Gout.* Gout occurs when the blood uric acid is too high. The uric acid crystals deposit in the joints, which causes painful swelling. The swelling can occur in any joint, but it most commonly occurs in the big toe. The high level of uric acid in the blood causes a higher urinary uric acid, making it more likely that a uric acid stone will form.

People who suffer from gout tend to consume a lot of animal protein. They are more likely to have uric acid stones than the general population, but, conversely, most uric acid stone formers do not have gout. This point is often misunderstood.

However, it is quite possible to form a uric acid stone without an unusually large amount of uric acid in the urine.

• *Idiopathic uric acid lithiasis.* One way that the kidneys excrete acid is by "binding" the acid onto a molecule of ammonia, making ammonium ions. The ammonium ions carry the acid out of the body. People with idiopathic uric acid lithiasis have a defect in the kidneys' ability to generate ammonia in response to an acid load. The urine of these patients is consistently acid, which predisposes them to stone formation. The effect of a urinary pH that remains close to 5.0 all of the time is more important than the absolute amount of uric acid in the urine.

• *Chronic diarrhea* and *ileostomies.* Both of these conditions lead to a chronic loss of fluid from the lower intestine. Lower intestinal fluid is alkaline. (See "Acid and Base" in Chapter 2.) Therefore, the loss leads to a correspondingly acid urine that makes uric acid stone formation likely. Furthermore, the loss of water leads to a reduction in urine volume that compounds the tendency to stone formation. People with ileostomies are at particular risk for uric acid stones because they have lower urinary volume and lower urinary pH than normal.

•   *Animal protein intake.*   Animal protein contains large amounts of purines, the uric acid precursors. Glandular meats, such as liver and sausages, are particularly high in purines, but all animal protein foods contain significant amounts of these uric acid sources.

Excess protein intake (the 16-ounce steak dinner or the whole chicken some people eat "because it was a small chicken") increases the amount of purine presented to the kidneys and thereby increases the amount of acid that must be excreted.

•   *Eating habits.*   Many patients with uric acid stones are binge eaters, or they participate in fasting or diet supplement programs for rapid weight loss. The sudden increase in dietary protein, or dieting with protein supplements, will tend to increase uric acid excretion. (See Chapter 10, "Dieting Your Way to a Kidney Stone.")

It is interesting to note that uric acid stones are more common in people over age fifty than calcium-containing stones. They are the one kind of stone whose incidence increases with age. The ability of the kidney to handle acids changes as we get older. And, in some people, the kidney cannot generate ammonia the way it should. Therefore, it never quite catches up with acid excretion. The pH of the urine stays acid, which predisposes these people to kidney stones.

Cystine Stones

Cystinuria is an uncommon genetic disorder that causes the kidney to excrete too much of the *amino acid* cystine in the urine. If there is too much cystine in the urine, it can form stones.

While people with cystinuria can make their first stones at almost any age, the disease should be suspected in anyone with a stone before the age of twenty. The disease is inherited as a recessive trait. That means that a child can have cystinuria even if neither parent has it. Many physicians will screen people with multiple stones for this disorder, particularly if the stones have not been caught for analysis.

Management of stone disease in people with cystinuria should be handled by a physician with a special interest in stone disease. This doctor will usually be a nephrologist or an endocrinologist. (See Chapter 23, "Choosing a Specialist.")

Struvite Stones

Struvite, or infected, stones are among the most difficult and dangerous problems in stone disease because of the potential of life-threatening complications from infection. These stones are found mainly
in women with recurring urinary infections, paralyzed patients, and
patients with abnormal urinary tracts. They are infection-related and
they frequently complicate other types of stones. Struvite stones are
often called *triple phosphate stones* because they contain three different elements: magnesium, ammonium, and calcium.

These stones tend to recur and are difficult to remove. People
with struvite stones suffer from frequent episodes of *pyelonephritis*
(kidney infections), renal obstruction, and a backflow of infected urine
into the bloodstream, which can be life threatening. This is one
important reason physicians look for fever during any stone episode.

Struvite stones are caused by certain bacteria, the most common
of which is called *Proteus.* An established or persistent urinary infection can generate this special type of stone material.

When a urinary infection occurs in a patient with preexisting
stones, struvite can be layered on top of the original stone. There can
be a core of calcium oxalate or uric acid and an outer shell of struvite.

While calcium oxalate stones are well-organized crystals, struvite
stones are quite amorphous, like lava. They spread out inside the
kidney and form to the branched shape of the collecting system. (See
Figure 1, page 11.) When this happens, the branching appearance of
the stone looks like the antlers of a male deer. Hence, these stones are
sometimes called *staghorn calculi.* Struvite stones can clog up the
entire collecting system.

Complications of Other Stones with Struvite

Since struvite can layer itself on other kinds of stones, it presents
special complications. These often occur in patients with urinary tract
infections (primarily women), paralyzed patients with impaired bladder function, catheterized patients, and patients with dysfunctional
or anatomically abnormal urinary tracts.

A small calcium oxalate stone that becomes infected with *Proteus* can then grow into a huge staghorn calculus that blocks up and
destroys an entire kidney.

Children with Struvite Stones

The most common cause of kidney stones in children is an inherited abnormality in the urinary tract that predisposes them to infection. Therefore, struvite stones represent a much larger fraction of stones in children than in adults.

Treatment for struvite stones consists of eliminating the organism causing the infection, or inhibiting the enzyme that generates the chemical conditions causing the stone. Antibiotics, control of dietary phosphate and protein intake, aluminum hydroxide, and removal of the stone(s) may be necessary to protect the kidney.

Bladder Stones

Although a protein-rich diet is at the heart of the stone epidemic in Western countries, bladder stones occur in young male children of underdeveloped countries primarily as the result of malnutrition. In Western countries, bladder stones are usually an indication of some kind of lower urinary tract obstruction. In the 1800s in Europe, there were large numbers of bladder stones. As the Industrial Revolution took place and Europe became more affluent, the incidence of bladder stones went down dramatically. The major peak in the incidence of bladder stones in children younger than ten is now seen in Asia. We can trace this incidence directly to poor protein intake and a lack of adequate dietary phosphorus. When children have milk, the incidence of bladder stones disappears.

Bladder stones are more common in men, especially those with prostatic obstructions or with urethral strictures from previous venereal disease such as *gonorrhea* (see Chapter 11). When they occur in women, which is uncommon, they are usually due to bladder dysfunction from a neurological disease that causes abnormal bladder emptying.

Importance of Stone Analysis

The exact composition of a stone gives your doctor an important clue as to the reasons why the stone has formed. This information may not be available from any other type of workup. As we discussed, a calcium-containing stone that has a mineral called carbonate apatite may indicate the presence of renal tubular acidosis (RTA). It is important for the treating physician to have this information, as RTA is treated quite differently from other causes of stone disease. (See "Rental Tubular Acidosis" in Chapter 9.)

If I find a small amount of struvite, I know that infection has played a role. If I find cystine in a stone, the information tells me you have cystinuria, even if other minerals are present. If I find uric acid in a calcium oxalate stone, I know that I must treat for both problems.

Kidney stones come in many different sizes, shapes, and, most importantly, compositions. Each stone type has its own causes, complicating factors, and dietary emphasis.

5

HOW AND WHY
KIDNEY STONES FORM

*My mother has a terrible stomach. My father had an even
worse stomach. The combination of their genes caused my
sister and myself. Sometimes I'll drink a glass of water
and get intense heartburn from the water.*

Your chances of forming kidney stones are largely determined by
your genetic makeup and by the way your diet and lifestyle interplay
with this genetic inheritance.

Genetics

If one or both of your parents made stones, there is a greater chance
that you will make stones. But your diet and fluid intake make a big
difference in whether or not the gene that controls stone formation
can assert itself. This situation is similar to high cholesterol—which
also runs in families—where a strict diet can make a huge difference
in the likelihood of cardiovascular disease.

Diet and Lifestyle

It is also possible to form stones even if it is not a part of your family
history. If you do so, it is probably a result of your diet or specific
lifestyle. For example, kidney stones often occur in people who move
to hot, dry climates and in people whose work or exercise causes
them to perspire heavily.

Whether you have a family history of stones or your stones are a result of a dietary or lifestyle change, if you want to stop kidney stones from forming, you must understand what to do to stop this process before it starts. You need to know the basic factors that encourage the formation of urinary crystals.

What Is a Kidney Stone?

A kidney stone consists of crystals that become organized into a large enough mass to be visible with the naked eye. In many cases, the stones contain more than one type of crystal, such as a combination of calcium oxalate and uric acid. But the crystals form a stone only when there are enough of them in the urine and the right conditions are present.

A simple way to understand the conditions that promote stone formation is to look at how rock candy is made.

The Rock Candy Principle

To make rock candy, we need three basic ingredients: 1 cup of water, 2 cups of sugar, and a string.

If we combine the water and sugar in a pot, a layer of sugar will sink to the bottom. If we then heat the mixture, the sugar dissolves. Chemists call this going into "solution," which means in this case that you can't see it, but you can taste it.

When the mixture is cooled slowly, the sugar stays in solution. We can take our string, dip it in the cooling pot, and candy crystals will form on the string. Two important things have happened to cause the candy to crystallize on the string.

First, by heating the water, we put more sugar into it than it would normally absorb, thereby making a supersaturated solution: There is more sugar in the water than can stay in solution for any period of time.

Second, we needed something to start the crystals forming. When we inserted the string into the solution, it acted as a "promoter."

That is exactly what happens in your urine: It becomes full of more of the things that make stones than it can hold onto. And certain promoters, such as the waste products of protein metabolism, encourage the formation of crystals, which grow into stones.

Discouraging Crystal Formation

If we wanted to discourage the formation of our rock candy "stone," we could

- Put less sugar in the pot.
- Pour more water in the pot and dilute the water so that the solution becomes undersaturated.
- Take away the string.

If you want to prevent kidney stones from forming, you must

- Eat less of the foods that form crystals.
- Drink more water to dilute the urine.
- Eliminate the foods and factors that promote stones.

Although analogies make it easier to understand urine chemistry, you must remember that kidney stones are not made of sugar and are not triggered by strings but by chemical wastes in the urine.

What Kidney Stones Are Made Of

Stones can be composed of either single substances or salts, which are two or more substances that join together. Uric acid and cystine are single substances. On the other hand, calcium stones and struvite stones are each composed of salts.

Salts

Salts have two parts. One side, with a positive charge, is the cation; the other side, with a negative charge, is the anion. Together they make a salt. We can describe salts as the chemical version of the term "opposites attract."

For example, table salt is sodium and chloride. Baking soda, which you use to keep your refrigerator from smelling, is sodium and bicarbonate. The solution put on tennis courts to make them smooth is a salt: calcium and chloride. The important fact to remember about salts is that they are brought together by their positive and negative charges.

Calcium Oxalate Salts

We are interested here in one particular salt—calcium oxalate—because it makes up the vast majority of kidney stones. Calcium is the cation and oxalate is the anion; they come together to make kidney stones. Calcium oxalate is a very insoluble salt, which means that it takes very little calcium and oxalate together in solution to form crystals.

Since the body is usually getting rid of more of these minerals than the urine can hold, your urine is often in a position where it is primed to make crystals.

The Conditions That Favor Crystal Formation

The likelihood of a person forming calcium oxalate stones depends, first of all, on how much calcium and how much oxalate is present. Because the ratio of calcium to oxalate is usually around 10 to 1, small changes in the amount of oxalate in the urine actually have a greater effect on the potential of urine to form stones than do small changes in the amount of calcium.

There are also promoters in the urine such as monosodium urate, which is a form of uric acid. The crystal structure of monosodium urate and calcium oxalate is very similar. Monosodium urate can "seed" the growth of a calcium oxalate crystal. More urate therefore means the urine is more likely to make a calcium oxalate stone.

The Best Inhibitor of Kidney Stones

If urine is often supersaturated with respect to calcium oxalate, why isn't everyone making stones all the time? The reason is that urine also contains inhibitors that keep calcium oxalate in solution. There is no convenient analogy in the rock candy model, but the idea of an inhibitor is easy to understand.

Citrate is the body's best inhibitor of kidney stones. The more citrate in your urine, the less likely you are to form a calcium oxalate crystal.

Urine Component	Stone Risk
Calcium ↑	↑
Oxalate ↑	↑
Urate ↑	↑
Volume ↑	⇩
Citrate ↑	⇩

Figure 3.   Risk Factors for Calcium Oxalate Stones
When there is an increase of calcium, oxalate, and/or urate in the urine, the risk of forming a calcium oxalate stone increases. Conversely, an increase in the volume of urine or citrate decreases the risk of stone disease.

The vast majority of citrate is made right in the kidney and controlled by urinary pH. (See the section on pH, "Acid and Base," in Chapter 3.) The kidney makes more citrate if urinary pH is high (alkaline) and less if it is low (acidic). The only function of citrate seems to be to control the formation of stones.

Finally, the more dilute a urine is, the less likely it is to make a calcium oxalate crystal.

It is possible to assess the risk of forming a calcium oxalate stone by considering the makeup of your urine. (See Figure 3.)

Making a Uric Acid Stone

Unlike calcium oxalate, which is a salt, uric acid is a single substance and exists in two forms: uric acid itself and urate. The urate is much more soluble. As the pH of the urine rises from 5.0 to 7.0, more of the uric acid is converted into urate. (See "Acid and Base" in Chapter 3.) The solubility is eleven times higher at pH 7.0 than it is at pH 5.0. Therefore, in an acid urine, uric acid crystals can form and grow into a stone. As the pH rises, uric acid stones can dissolve.

The urate form of uric acid can also promote the formation of calcium oxalate stones.

Therefore, an increase in the amount of uric acid in the urine makes both uric acid and calcium oxalate stones more likely. The risk of developing a uric acid stone can be assessed by considering:

Total uric acid excreted
Urinary pH profile (see Chapter 13, "The Workup")
How concentrated the urine is

Understanding how stones form enables you to understand why we must manipulate certain elements in your urine to stop this process.

6

WHY KIDNEY STONES ARE SO PAINFUL

The first time was like a living death. You can't lie down, you can't sit down, you just roll around on the floor. On the way to the doctor's, I had to pull over on the parkway and roll out of the car. You want to die.

After watching two children being born, it's really not that different. Emotionally, of course, it's not as good in the end. The only consolation is that I didn't have to buy a savings bond after I passed my stones.

I've been in car accidents that weren't as painful as passing a stone.

Stones may lie silently in the kidney for years. But when a stone passes into and obstructs the ureter—the narrow tube connecting the kidney to the bladder—excruciating pain usually follows. The pain may stop as suddenly as it occurred when the stone passes into the bladder.

The kind of pain you have depends on the location of the stone. Not all kidney stones cause pain; some are discovered only by X ray.

Kinds of Pain

There are two kinds of pain people experience when passing stones.

34

Soreness of the Kidney

When a stone is passing, the kidney can swell. This irritates the nerves in the capsule surrounding the kidney (the *renal capsule*), causing soreness. The kidney or flank becomes tender to the touch because it is swollen.

This swelling of the kidney and the surrounding kidney capsule makes it painful to walk around. If you were riding in a car and went over a bump, you might have tenderness.

People can also experience a sore flank during physical activity. This can be caused by the sharp, hard object (the stone) rattling around in the soft tissue of the kidney, basically punching it.

But the "agony" that people describe has nothing to do with the kidney being swollen.

Colic

> *I couldn't sit. I couldn't stand. I couldn't lie down. I've broken numerous bones in my life and I would say it's right up there.*

The big pain occurs when the muscle inside the ureter is trying to work the stone down and out.

Muscles are designed to move things in the body. There are three basic types of muscle: cardiac, skeletal, and smooth. *Cardiac muscle* moves blood in and out of your heart and is found only in that organ. *Skeletal muscle* moves *you* around and controls the voluntary movements of your arms, legs, chest, and so on. *Smooth muscle* moves things around your inner organs and blood vessels. It lines the uterus, bile ducts, blood vessels, intestines, and the urinary tract. The contractions of smooth muscle are involuntary.

When smooth muscle goes into spasm, it is called *colic*. This occurs when smooth muscle is working against a blockage or obstruction, and colic *hurts*.

Most people are familiar with some type of smooth muscle spasm. The colicky baby cries in pain as the smooth muscle tries to move gas out of the intestine. The main pain women experience during labor is the smooth muscle spasm of the uterus as it moves the baby out. The spasm that occurs when the smooth muscle inside the ureter is trying to work a kidney stone down and out is called *renal colic*.

The Six Great Pains of Medicine

The six great pains of medicine are heart attack, angleclosure glaucoma (acute closure of the drainage angle of the eye, leading to increased pressure), tic douloureux (facial nerve pain), childbirth, biliary colic (passing a gallbladder stone), and renal colic (passing a kidney stone). Three of these six pains are colics. Many people think that renal colic is the most severe of them all.

When you have bad colic, there is no way to make yourself comfortable. Most people choose to pace up and down.

There are three basic renal colic pain patterns. The kind of renal colic you have depends on where the stone is. (See Figure 4.)

1. *Ureteropelvic stone.*   If the stone is in the pelvis of the kidney or upper ureter, you may feel the pain in your flank. Men sometimes feel the pain in the testicle on the same side as the kidney stone, even though there is nothing wrong with the testicle. This referred pain has its explanation in the development of the male urinary tract. The ducts that drain the kidney and the testicle in the male fetus come from a similar embryological origin. Therefore, the adult male may perceive a spasm in the pelvis of the kidney as pain in the testicle. It is somewhat like a crossed circuit.

2. *Midureteral stone.*   As the stone starts to move down the ureter, the pain moves a little bit toward the front and radiates down to the groin. Men will not feel it in the testicle anymore.

3. *Low ureteral stone.*   When the stone reaches the bladder tunnel, the pain radiates down toward the scrotum in the male or vulva in the female. People develop what is called *vesicle irritability*, the vesicle being the medical term for bladder.

When the bladder is irritated, people may suddenly feel a tremendous urge to urinate even though the bladder has just been emptied. And, even if you go to urinate, you'll keep feeling this urge, no matter how much urine you pass. Another example of a crossed circuit, this sensation occurs because the trigone, the part of the bladder that gives you the sensation of voiding, is irritated by the stone. (See Chapter 2, Figure 1.) This irritation sends the "I need to urinate" signal, even though no urine may be present. A woman with an acute bladder infection may also experience this false signal when the trigone is inflamed.

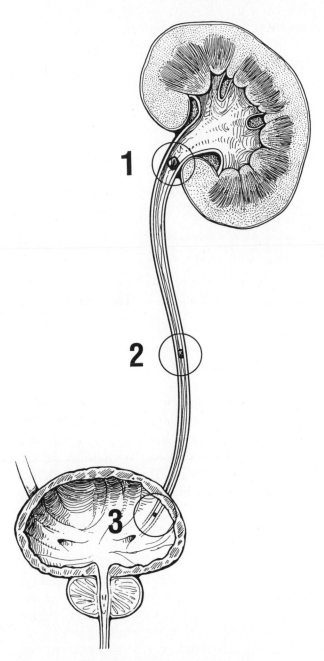

Figure 4.   Where Kidney Stones Hang Up
The pain patterns are different for stones in each of these three places.

When the stone finally, and often quite suddenly, pops into your bladder, you feel the most unbelievable sense of relief because the smooth muscle stops its spasms. There may be some burning on urination when the stone passes through the *urethra*, but the pain is rarely as severe, for the urethra is much bigger and hardly ever goes into spasm.

Ball-valve Situation

Sometimes the stone may move into the upper ureter and then bounce back into the kidney. This "ball-valve situation" may produce intermittent soreness and/or colic.

People may experience both soreness and colic, and they may come together. Interestingly, some of the worse pain comes from the smallest stones—often the size of a grain of sand—as opposed to the bigger stones. We do not really understand why.

Three Areas in the Kidney Where Stones Hang Up

There may be relief during a stone episode if the stone stops moving. But the mere fact that the pain has stopped does not mean that the stone has passed. I have seen patients who begin to pass a stone and then have the stone stop. A month or two later, we find that there is actually a stone stuck in the urinary tract. This is one situation to watch carefully because the obstruction caused by the stone may damage the kidney.

Figure 4 (page 37) shows the three common places where stones can stop moving.

1. *Pelvis of kidney.*   This occurs particularly when the junction of the ureter is somewhat narrowed.
2. *Iliac artery/branch of aorta.*   Stoppage here can occur because the ureter makes a little curve over this large blood vessel.
3. *Bladder tunnel.*   When a stone is hung up in the bladder tunnel, patients are left with an annoying urge to void that can be as disturbing as pain.

When a stone does not pass, it is time to call the Urologist. (See Chapter 23, "Choosing a Specialist.")

Secondary Symptoms

Many people with colic develop secondary symptoms including fever, nausea, and vomiting. These secondary symptoms can be quite important and may indicate the need for hospitalization.

Vomiting

During an episode of renal colic, the ability to keep fluids down is crucial. An increased urinary output is needed to wash the stone down so that it will pass unassisted. If you are unable to drink enough fluids, or if you become dehydrated from vomiting, you may need to be hospitalized and given intravenous fluids.

Fever and Chills

The second thing to watch for is fever. This may indicate an infection behind the stone. The infection has no place to go and can potentially spill into the bloodstream. We call this situation *sepsis*, and it is potentially fatal. For this reason physicians tell people who are passing a stone to monitor their temperature and to report fever. If fever does occur, it is potentially a medical emergency.

Chills can also represent incipient fever. A temperature of 100°F. or shaking chills during stone passage requires at least an urgent consultation with your doctor.

People with diabetes, prior urinary tract infections, kidney cysts, sickle cell anemia, prior urinary tract surgery or cystoscopy, abnormal urinary tract anatomy, and paralysis are more likely than others to get into trouble with infection while passing stones.

Blood in the Urine

When you pass a stone, you will often find blood in the urine, because most stones have rough edges that tear the urinary tract.

Calcium oxalate stones are often called *jackstones* because their sharp crystalline spikes look like those seen on a child's toy jacks.

If you already know that you are passing a stone and your urine is intermittently pink, you are probably all right unless other symptoms are also occurring. Physicians worry about blood in the urine when someone is producing clots that could cause obstruction, or when the amount of blood coming out represents significant blood loss. This is not usually the case during stone passage. While any blood in the urine can be scary, it is not often very serious. A tiny drop of blood can color a pint of urine pink. It takes only a little more to make it red.

Nevertheless, if you see blood in your urine, tell your doctor. There are no exceptions to this rule.

Never Make Your Own Diagnosis of a Stone

This book cannot anticipate all clinical situations. I saw one patient who had passed two kidney stones and, a year later, developed an episode with blood in the urine. It turned out that the blood in the urine was coming from a tumor in the kidney. If this person had assumed that this was another stone episode, a very serious problem would have been missed.

Treating Pain

I told the doctor: fix me or shoot me.

The most important aspect of pain management is to determine if you are actually passing a kidney stone. There is a danger that you will take, or be given, pain medication to alleviate renal colic and not be aware of another problem that requires urgent medical attention.

For example, I saw one patient who had passed several stones who then developed right-sided abdominal pain. Even though the pain was of a different quality, he assumed it came from another stone. He was about twelve hours late in coming to the emergency room for appendicitis. Fortunately, he had no long-term complications, but the potential for a disaster was there.

The decision to take pain medication for what you believe is a stone episode is yours and your physician's and should not be undertaken without proper consultation.

Generally, *acetaminophen* (not aspirin or ibuprofen) is used for mild pain; acetaminophen with codeine (e.g., Tylenol 3) or hydrocodone for slightly stronger pain; and oxycodone or percocet for fairly severe colic.

Sometimes the colic is so severe that the pain cannot be managed with any of the medications available at home. Or a person may be vomiting or have extreme nausea and be unable to tolerate oral medication for pain. It is not at all unusual for people to have to seek injectable pain medication in the emergency room.

There is one final point to reinforce about the treatment of pain: When you are having an episode of renal colic and the pain stops, it does not necessarily mean that the stone is out. A stone stuck midureter can stop hurting, but it can eventually cause trouble to the kidney. *You should always consult a physician after a stone episode.* Having a stone in your hand does not mean that you do not have another stone upstream. They sometimes come in volleys.

When Hospitalization Is Needed

The most important part of the management of stone passage is maintaining your urine flow. Since the process of passing a stone can cause nausea and vomiting, you can become quite dehydrated. That means the kidneys will make very little urine and there will not be enough to push the stone out.

If you have a diarrheal episode and are passing a stone, you also need to think about hydration. If you cannot maintain your urine output, get to the emergency room.

If any of the following symptoms occur when you are passing a stone, you need to go to the hospital:

1. Inability to drink fluids
2. Repeated vomiting
3. Fever
4. Unmanageable pain

Please note: This information is given with the assumption that there is no question as to your diagnosis. *Do not assume that you are passing a stone.* If you are not sure, call your physician.

7

HOW MUCH WATER DO I REALLY HAVE TO DRINK?

Don't tell the doctor, but I don't drink as much water as he told me to. I can't—I teach all day. I can't leave the classroom every half hour to go to the bathroom.

I feel as if I have to stay home in order to drink that amount of water and to be by a bathroom. I can't have a life.

Drinking that much is annoying as hell. I really should be wearing a diaper.

Fluids are the single most important ingredient in the prevention of kidney stones. There is no way to overestimate their importance. Theoretically, you could eat anything you wanted to and never make a stone if you drank enough. If you have a low urinary volume, nothing in this book is more important than getting you to drink more.

Causes of Low Urinary Output

Urine volume may be low for many reasons. The most obvious is not drinking enough fluids. Less obvious are work and lifestyle routines that cause dehydration.

A change in exercise regimes can leave you unexpectedly dehydrated. New joggers sometimes jog their way to a stone when they do not increase their fluid intake appropriately.

Hot summer weather causes dehydration. British doctors looked at soldiers arriving in the Persian Gulf for duty in May and November. They found five times more stones in the May arrivals than in the November group.

Some people have diarrheal losses of fluid. Others have occupations that make it inconvenient for them to drink or urinate (e.g., teachers and construction workers) so they habitually avoid drinking. (See "The Balance Concept" in Chapter 2, and Chapter 16, "Lifestyles of the Kidney Stone Former.")

A few women have been taught that it is "unladylike" to urinate, so they are psychologically conditioned to limit their fluid intake.

Travelers may be afraid of the local water supply. If their travels take them to tropical climates, dehydration can be the cause of their stones.

How Much Is Enough?

Many of my patients ask me: "How much do I have to drink?" My answer is always the same. Enough. Enough to produce a urinary volume of 2000 cc—roughly 2 quarts or 2 liters per day, or eight 8-ounce glasses of water—and preferably more. Unfortunately, it is not always practical or acceptable to maintain a urine volume over 2 liters.

So, we have to be practical. The teacher who cannot leave the classroom should drink two or three glasses of water before lunch and have the whole lunch hour to process the water and pass this fluid as urine. Fluids should be consumed again when arriving home to make up for the daytime lack.

Since it is impossible to predict nonurine fluid losses, the emphasis is on what comes out, not on what goes in. "Eight 8-ounce glasses of water daily" will be enough for a sedentary office worker in the wintertime, but it will leave the same person far short of the therapeutic goal if this person spends summers at the beach or out-of-doors.

Hard Water, Soft Water

There are conflicting data on the effect of hard tap water on stone incidence. One would expect that more calcium in the drinking water would increase urinary calcium, particularly in people with absorptive hypercalciuria. I have treated patients whose stone-forming prospensity decreased when they installed a water softener at home.

However, there are epidemiological data that suggest that fewer stones are formed in communities where the water is hard than in those with naturally soft water. There are several possible explanations. First, hard water has magnesium, which is a mild inhibitor of stones. Second, preparation of high-oxalate foods with hard water removes a lot of oxalate during the cooking. Therefore, these patients may not absorb as much oxalate, a major component in most stones.

There is no final word on this issue. We must be careful with epidemiological data when deciding what is best for a given person.

If your water supply is very hard and you need a softening system to save your household plumbing, by all means do it. Hard water tastes bad. Drinking water is important, so do all you can to make it taste good. Mildly hard water is probably harmless unless you suffer from severe absorptive hypercalciuria. (See Chapter 3.)

Mineral Water

Mineral water is often overlooked as a contributing factor to stone formation. Naturally carbonated water acquires its carbonation from dissolved limestone and, therefore, has a high calcium content. Artificially carbonated beverages get their carbonation from gas that is forced into the liquid under pressure.

People who drink bottled water should avoid large amounts of naturally carbonated water, particularly if they have hypercalciuria. Nongaseous bottled water may or may not have as high a calcium content as the naturally carbonated varieties.

How to Consume More Water

Because increasing your water intake is so critical to the treatment and elimination of kidney stones, we offer several suggestions to help you consume more water. You can probably expand this list.

- Drink a full glass of water before you brush your teeth in the morning and another glass with breakfast.

- Drink one to two glasses of water with every meal and, if you can, with your midmorning or midafternoon snack or break.
- Eat foods with a high water content, for example, jello or watermelon.
- Drink a glass of water when you get home at night and another before dinner. This fluid should pass long before you go to bed and not interrupt a good night's sleep.
- Drink a glass of water before going to sleep and keep one by your bed. This is especially important for people with cystinuria and for other severe stone formers. Waking up in the middle of the night to urinate is not nearly as painful as waking up with renal colic.

  People with cystinuria and other severe stone disease problems must put up with increased urine flow at night if they are going to minimize stone formation. This is one of the most difficult aspects of stone control for these people.
- Sip water during the day. Keep water on your desk if you are in an office, in a covered container in the car, and in a thermos when you are outdoors. Sip.
- Put up a sign on your refrigerator or bathroom mirror: Drink an Extra Glass of Water Today.

The Role of Fluids

I know we've said this before, but it is important enough to mention it again. A high urinary output is the most important part of kidney stone management. We will repeat this throughout this book, and you should post a reminder to drink extra fluids on your refrigerator door. When you arrive in the kitchen for dinner or that late-night snack, wash it down and out with an extra glass of water.

8

DIETARY TROUBLEMAKERS

I need a "hit" list: These are foods to avoid, these are acceptable, these are foods that are good for you.

After fluids, there are four major dietary "danger" substances that affect stone formers dramatically: protein, calcium, oxalates, and salt. The effects of certain vitamin supplements and alcohol consumption are also important.

Although we focus here on specific dietary troublemakers, you must remember that everything you eat counts: the water you drink or don't drink from a water fountain you pass at work; that piece of chocolate candy you surreptitiously take from the desk of an officemate; the occasional "cheat" that starts to happen regularly. Everything you eat counts and affects the formation of kidney stones.

How Much You Eat Is Just as Important as What You Eat

When patients ask me for a "hit list" of foods to avoid, I tell them that there is a list of foods high in certain stone-forming elements (see the food charts in the Appendix), but they must consider "how much" they eat as well as "what."

For example, tomatoes are a moderate oxalate food. Oxalate is a component, with calcium, of the majority of kidney stones. (See Chapter 4.) You will not make a stone if you put a slice of tomato into your salad every so often. But the process of making a tomato *sauce* concentrates the amount of oxalate found in the tomato. A single $1/_2$ cup of tomato sauce may contain the oxalate of ten tomatoes. Therefore, if you eat tomato sauce in large quantities, your oxalate

46

burden is going to be considerable. You must look at the *quantity* of certain foods that you eat, as well as the level of stone-forming elements in those foods.

Animal Protein Is Animal Protein

You must reduce the portion size of *all kinds of meat* including chicken, veal, and fish. White meat is still meat.

I often ask patients: "How much meat do you eat?" And they reply: "very little." It then turns out that they are consuming enormous portions of chicken and turkey. For the purposes of stone formation, these meats are just as bad as red meat.

If you have a high cholesterol and must control your fat intake, the substitution of chicken and fish for red meat may be beneficial. (Note: Remember to take off the skin.) If you have kidney stones, *all* animal protein is the same. (See the Appendix, Tables 5 and 6.)

Protein and Kidney Stones

After low urinary volume, a high animal protein intake is the most important factor influencing the frequency of kidney stone disease.

Protein is the essential building block of all body tissues. It is necessary for

- The building and repair of various body tissues
- Energy
- The structure of enzymes, hormones, and various fluids and body secretions
- Forming antibodies in the immune system, as well as other substances that transport minerals and vitamins to the body

However, eating too much animal protein increases the risk of stone formation.

The Problem with Animal Protein

Diets high in animal protein will increase the chance of forming both uric acid and calcium oxalate stones for three related but slightly different reasons (see also Chapter 5):

1. Animal protein contains large amounts of a substance called purines, whose end product is uric acid. More uric acid in the urine means that you are more likely to make a uric acid stone. In addition, one form of uric acid, urate, can act as a seed for calcium oxalate stones.
2. The excessive consumption of animal protein will lower the pH of urine, making it more acid (See "Acid and Base" in Chapter 3.) This lower urinary pH makes uric acid less soluable and thereby favors the formation of uric acid stones. It also suppresses citrate formation by the kidney, which reduces one of the body's natural inhibitors of calcium oxalate formation.
3. One of the amino acids in all proteins, glycine, is metabolized to oxalate. Another amino acid, methionine, drives out more calcium in the urine. A diet higher in protein will therefore increase urinary calcium even though the amount of calcium in the diet remains constant.

Therefore, both uric acid stone formers and calcium oxalate stone formers must learn to control animal protein portions. Meat consumption in the industrialized nations is currently at an all-time high. Although the consumption of *red* meat is considerably lower than in past years, we have replaced it with very ample servings of chicken and fish.

Watch Your Portion Size

The best approach to animal protein is to reduce the portion size of all meat in your diet. The recommended portion for any meat is about 3 ounces. This is approximately the size of a deck of cards. Eating less meat may also reduce your total caloric intake and help you lose weight, if that is a secondary goal.

The Calcium Controversy

Calcium is the most abundant mineral in the body, and it performs many functions (see also Chapters 14 and 15):

• It is the raw material for the growth of bones and teeth.
• It stimulates muscle contraction.

- It stimulates blood clotting.
- It assists in the transmission of nerve impulses.

Adequate calcium intake throughout life helps prevent *osteoporosis* (weak bones), and researchers have found a possible link between low calcium intake and elevated blood pressure.

Calcium is found in dairy foods and many nondairy foods that are also high in oxalate, such as kale and spinach. (See the Appendix.)

Calcium is also the most abundant mineral in kidney stones.

Calcium Issues

Calcium stone formers generally have a high urinary calcium. If you increase dietary calcium in a normal person, you will have a slightly elevated urinary calcium. Therefore, the traditional recommendation for calcium stone formers has been a low-calcium diet.

There are several reasons for being cautious about such a recommendation.

- *Bone Density.* There is evidence to indicate that stone formers as a group have lower bone densities than the general population. If you are on a low-calcium diet, your bone problem is going to get worse, particularly as you grow older.

In addition to the risk of a decreased mineral content of bone, a very low-calcium diet places many patients with hypercalciuria in negative calcium balance. This means that the body, as a whole, is losing calcium.

- *Increased Urinary Oxalate.* A low-calcium diet may also allow the body to increase its absorption of oxalates.

Ordinarily, there is an excess of calcium over oxalate in the first part of your intestine. Since calcium and oxalate combine easily, most of the oxalate in your diet unites with calcium in the upper intestine. In essence, tiny calcium oxalate stones form inside your bowel. Since the intestine is so wide, these tiny stones make no difference. There is, however, very little oxalate available as your food moves to the last part of the intestine, the colon. And it is in the colon that most oxalate is absorbed by the body.

In other words, with ordinary bowel function, only a very small part of the ingested oxalate is absorbed because most of it combines with calcium in the first part of the intestine.

This explains one of the problems with a very low-calcium diet. If there is too little calcium in the first part of the intestine, more oxalate will remain free inside the intestine, and more oxalate will be absorbed. It is one reason why rigid dietary calcium restriction is not recommended for most stone formers. Although urinary calcium may drop, the excessive absorption of oxalate in the intestine can actually aggravate a stone-forming problem.

In a recent study, men over age forty on low-calcium diets made *more* stones than men on medium-calcium diets. The increased oxalate absorption may have been a factor.

 •   *Replacing Dairy Products with High-Oxalate Foods*.   I have found that people often replace dairy products with foods high in oxalate or its precursors. People advised to consume less milk, cheese, and ice cream may then eat more nuts, chocolate, and fruit juices.

Calcium Guidelines

It is hard to write calcium guidelines for all stone formers. Generally, I would limit the person drinking 2 quarts of milk a day but caution people that avoiding all calcium-containing foods is equally bad. The specific amounts of calcium a stone former should consume depend on urinary chemistries (see Chapter 13), the incidence or risk of osteoporosis, and the patient's condition.

The amount of calcium recommended for a stone former may be the most controversial topic in this book. If you have had a serious stone problem, there is no substitute for having your urinary calcium measured. You should also have a "calcium loading test" to determine the percentage of calcium your body absorbs. If tests show that you have absorptive hypercalciuria, a condition in which the intestine overabsorbs calcium, it will be more important to control your dairy product intake.

When I do not have a measurement of urinary calcium to guide my recommendations, I generally advise stone formers to consume the equivalent of an 8-ounce glass of milk daily. The aim is to be on neither a high- nor a low-calcium diet.

Consult your physician for an exact dietary prescription for calcium.

Calcium Supplements

Many people are now taking calcium supplements to retard the development of osteoporosis. Some physicians have expressed a fear that such supplements are going to cause an epidemic of kidney stones. So far, that epidemic has not appeared, and calcium supplements have probably saved many postmenopausal women from spinal and hip fractures.

The problem is that some people assume that because some is good, more is better. They engage in unrestricted use of these supplements. Others take calcium supplements along with too much vitamin D, which enhances calcium absorption from the intestine. (See "Vitamins and Kidney Stones," this chapter.)

Until there are conclusive data regarding the stone-forming potential of calcium supplements in the general public, I advise any woman who has made stones and is considering calcium supplements for osteoporosis to discuss this supplement with her doctor. (See Chapter 24, "Medications.")

However, factors other than the ingestion of calcium may have an overriding effect on calcium excretion.

Salt

The mineral sodium (salt) is present in the body in comparatively large amounts. It occurs in greatest concentration in the fluid compartments surrounding cells and on the surface of bone.

Sodium has numerous functions in the body. It is involved in

- The normal water balance of the body
- Muscle contraction and expansion and in nerve stimulation
- The acid-base balance in the blood
- Regulation of blood pressure and blood volume

There are many sources of sodium in food (see the Appendix, Table 4) and especially in prepared products such as baked goods, cereals, and canned foods. Baking powder, baking soda, some preservatives, artificial sweeteners, and seasoning salts such as monosodium glutamate contain sodium. Toothpaste is high in sodium. And some drugs are also available as sodium salts.

Salt is often forgotten in the diet prescribed for the stone former. By itself, the sodium in your diet has only a minimal effect on the tendency of the urine to make stones. *However, an increase in dietary sodium increases the urinary calcium.* In other words, the more salt in your diet, the more calcium appears in your urine, even if your dietary calcium stays the same.

For example, if a patient consumes 900 milligrams of calcium and 100 milliequivalents of sodium, the urine calcium might be 200 milligrams in twenty-four hours. If a person consumes the same 900 milligrams of calcium but doubles his or her sodium intake to 200 milliequivalents, the urinary calcium could be as high as 350 milligrams in twenty-four hours.

This rise occurs because sodium affects the way your kidneys handle calcium, causing them to excrete more calcium. Therefore, the amount of salt a stone former consumes becomes more important.

Furthermore, if you are taking a thiazide diuretic to lower calcium (see Chapter 24), the thiazide will not lower your urinary calcium unless you control your salt intake. A decreased serum potassium, one of the side effects of thiazide diuretics, is also increased on a high-salt diet. (See Chapter 24, "Medications.")

Do not put yourself on a low-salt diet without consulting your physician. The best way to ascertain whether your salt consumption is excessive is to have your physician measure how much sodium comes out in your urine during a twenty-four-hour period.

Oxalate

Oxalate would be of little or no interest if it did not crystallize with calcium to form kidney stones. (See Chapter 4 on oxalate stones and Chapter 17, "Operation Oxalate.") In fact, oxalate is present in more than 75 percent of all stones. It comes from food, the metabolism of protein, the degradation of vitamin C, and general metabolism.

High-Oxalate Foods

Although the oxalate levels of different foods are difficult to measure accurately, there are certainly seven foods that greatly enhance urinary oxalate excretion. These are spinach, rhubarb, beets, nuts, chocolate, tea, and wheat bran. However, the "bioavailability" of the oxalate may be different in various foods. In other words, some oxalate-containing foods are more problematic than others. In various food tests, spinach seems to produce the greatest rise in urinary oxalate.

You remember the sailor: I thought spinach was a health food.

Patients with calcium oxalate stones must watch their oxalate intakes. One patient had taken the Popeye cartoon seriously and thought he would grow bigger and stronger if he ate a lot of spinach. The only thing that grew big was a kidney stone.

Some patients consume very large amounts of strong tea (or iced tea in the summer). Their dietary oxalate load from this drink may be considerable. I had a patient who started to keep a large pitcher of iced tea on his desk at work. He was consuming four to six large glasses a day. He formed his first stone two months later.

Since each person absorbs and excretes various dietary elements differently, a possible course of treatment is to measure oxalate excretion on and off tea consumption to see if there is a difference.

Some researchers have suggested that increases in urinary oxalate excretion may be more important than increases in urinary calcium in causing calcium oxalate stone disease. It is clear that oxalate metabolism has received less attention than calcium metabolism largely because the former is so difficult to measure.

I sometimes see patients who indulge in oxalate gluttony, particularly with seasonal foods. Iced tea in the summer, hot cocoa in the winter, and beefsteak tomatoes in September are a few examples. Spinach and other dark green, leafy vegetables, rhubarb, and even nuts, chocolate, and tea should be avoided. (See the Appendix, Table 2.) In Chapter 17, "Operation Oxalate," we will discuss control of dietary oxalate in more detail.

Vitamins and Kidney Stones

Each of the vitamins serves a different purpose in the human body.

Vitamin D

Vitamin D is needed to

- Prevent rickets
- Aid in the absorption of calcium and phosphorus from the intestine
- Keep bones healthy
- Promote dental health and growth

Vitamin D is found in both animal and plant sources. The richest sources are the fish-liver oils, eggs, liver, certain fish, and fortified milk products.

Since vitamin D is needed for growth, infants, children, and pregnant and lactating women need a daily intake of 400 IU (international units). Normal adults have minimal needs for vitamin D. Sunlight and small amounts from food sources are sufficient for adults to meet requirements.

Some older patients and women with osteoporosis may, under certain circumstances, benefit from taking supplements of vitamin D.

However, taken in excess, vitamin D can cause stone formation. Occasionally, someone who is taking too much vitamin D to "make better bones" overabsorbs calcium, becomes hypercalciuric, and makes stones. If a stone former consumes the recommended two to three servings of milk products daily and has a usual amount of exposure to sunlight, it is unlikely that supplemental vitamin D is needed.

I occasionally see vitamin D–toxic patients. One woman was taking steroids to control her asthma, and was given vitamin D to prevent bone disease. (Steroids may increase a tendency to osteoporosis.) When she no longer needed the steroids for her asthma, she kept taking the vitamin D and increased the dose. After her fourth stone she came to my office seeking an explanation for her numerous stones. While uncommon, vitamin D toxicity is one preventable cause of stone formation.

Vitamin D supplements are also given to people taking anticonvulsive medications such as Dilantin. (The anticonvulsives have been shown to interfere with vitamin D formation in the liver.) This situation must be handled carefully in order to avoid toxicity and the formation of stones. The supplement may be unnecessary if the seizure medication is discontinued.

Vitamin A

The body needs vitamin A for

* Vision
* Growth and reproduction
* Development and maintenance of epithelial tissue
* The immunity process

Vitamin A occurs in liver; whole and fortified milk; eggs; dark green, leafy vegetables such as spinach; and yellow-orange vegetables and fruit, such as carrots and squash. It occurs naturally in these foods as beta-carotene, which is metabolized by the body to vitamin A.

When the body does not need any more vitamin A, it stops metabolizing the beta-carotene. It is therefore difficult to get too much vitamin A from food. Kidney stone formers who restrict green leafy and yellow-orange vegetables due to their high oxalate content may benefit from beta-carotene supplements.

However, megadoses of vitamin A itself can lead to increased calcium excretion and liver toxicity. We are seeing more liver disease in people who take too much vitamin A. You should consult with your doctor before supplementing this vitamin.

Vitamin C

We need vitamin C to

* Prevent scurvy
* Enhance iron absorption
* Aid in wound healing
* Promote resistance to infection

Vitamin C is found in vegetables and fruits such as green and red peppers, collard greens, broccoli, spinach, tomatoes, potatoes, straw-berries, oranges, and other citrus fruits.

Excess amounts of vitamin C can be excreted in the urine as oxalate. Furthermore, vitamin C is an acid (ascorbic acid). It tends to lower urinary pH, which in turn lowers urinary citrate, a natural inhibitor of kidney stones (see Chapter 5).

Conclusions about the effect of dietary vitamin C on stone

formation have been contradictory. Some studies have suggested that increased vitamin C can raise the likelihood of stone formation, while others do not.

Until we have data proving that supplements of vitamin C can really provide protection against all the diseases that this vitamin is supposed to prevent, I advise my stone-forming patients not to take vitamin C supplements beyond what is in a balanced diet. For those who believe in vitamin C, I suggest you take no more than 500 milligrams a day. (See Chapter 10.)

Problems with Excessive Amounts of Vitamins

Vitamins occur naturally in foods. A well-balanced diet should provide all the vitamins needed by a healthy adult. Excessive supplements taken without the advice of your physician can lead to stone formation as well as other problems.

Alcohol

By itself, alcohol does not contribute to stone formation. However, it does have two effects that may set the stage for stone formation.

First, alcohol makes you pass more urine and can lead to dehydration. Second, alcohol indirectly inhibits the ability of the kidney to excrete uric acid. Here is a common scenario: You go to a steakhouse at 8 P.M. and start your dinner with a martini or two. You then have a large piece of roast beef with two beers or some wine. The alcohol dehydrates you and dams up the ability of the kidney to get rid of the uric acid. By 11 P.M. you have a huge backload of uric acid and other waste products from your meat meal. But your urine flow is reduced because your body has already passed an excessive amount of urine in response to the alcohol. This means that all of the stone-forming substances from the digestion of dinner come out in a very concentrated urine—setting up a perfect situation for stone formation.

In addition, there is a physiological process that slows urine flow while we are asleep, making it easier for us to sleep through the night. This slowed urinary flow, added to the dehydration from the martinis and beer, makes the urine very concentrated just at the time when it needs to be more dilute to deal with all of the waste products from dinner.

We will talk more about the issue of eating the largest, richest meal late in the day. (See Chapter 16, "Lifestyles of the Kidney Stone Former.") The tendency of more families to follow this late eating habit in the 1980s and 1990s may be one reason for the rising incidence of stone disease.

The Dietary Troublemakers

Remember, there are four major "hot spots" in a stone former's diet:

- Protein
- Calcium
- Oxalate
- Salt

They can all directly influence your potential for developing kidney stones, and they can interact with one another to tip the balance toward stone formation.

9

MEDICAL CONDITIONS THAT CAN CAUSE KIDNEY STONES

I had just gotten married and had to face surgery in the next month. I felt so sorry for myself. I had this thing hanging over my head on my honeymoon. I think I took it out on my husband.

—PATIENT WITH CYSTINURIA

I do some of my best work in the bathroom—I'm in there six to eight times a day.

—PATIENT WITH CROHN'S

It completely takes over your life: Everything is put on hold. You don't want to travel, you want to be near your doctor.

—PATIENT WITH HYPERCALCIURIA

There are a number of medical conditions that dispose people to the formation and recurrence of kidney stones. The twelve conditions described in this chapter are among the most common. While the diet and lifestyle advice given in this book is not designed to cure these underlying conditions, it can help control the formation of stones.

Bowel Disease

Often referred to as *inflammatory bowel disease*, this category includes conditions such as *colitis, Crohn's disease*, and *chronic diarrhea*.

People with bowel disease who do not absorb fluids and other nutrients normally may be predisposed to stone formation for three reasons:

* The loss of fluid leads to dehydration and a concentrated (stone-forming) urine.
* The loss of bicarbonate, or base, leads to an acid urine and the increased risk of uric acid stones; the acid urine also lowers urinary citrate, a natural inhibitor of calcium oxalate stone formation.
* Fat malabsorption prevents calcium from combining with oxalate in the first part of the intestine. Hence, more oxalate reaches the large intestine where it is absorbed, causing an increase in urinary oxalate.

Fluid Loss

As we explained in Chapter 3, the kidneys maintain a constant fluid balance in the body. The amount of fluid that comes out in the urine is equal to the amount consumed, minus losses from perspiration and the intestines. For people with bowel disease, this intestinal loss can be substantial.

When someone suffers from diarrhea, a great deal of fluid is lost through the intestines. The kidneys must then conserve fluid for the body. Therefore, the more diarrhea, the lower the urinary volume and the more concentrated the urine. And a concentrated urine means a greater concentration of stone-forming elements. (See Chapter 5.)

All people with bowel disease must be cautioned about fluid levels. The Ileitis and Colitis Foundation teaching pamphlets all emphasize this point.

Once again, we cannot tell you how much fluid to consume. The emphasis is not on the fluid you put in your mouth but on the urinary *output*. For people with bowel disease, this point is critical. Urinary output should stay above 2000 cc per day, preferably over 2500 cc.

Bicarbonate Loss

Lower gastrointestinal fluid is alkaline (basic). If the loss of alkali/bicarbonate is significant, the kidneys must make up for the loss of base by excreting a more acid urine. (See Chapter 3.)

Some people with ileostomies may lose several liters a day of alkaline fluid. They need to replace the fluid, but they may also need to put back the base lost. People with ileostomies should consult their physician regarding the need for base supplements to protect the body's acid/base balance.

If the urine is acid most, or all, of the time, you are at risk for making uric acid stones. Hence, anyone with an ileostomy or large daily losses of diarrhea will be at increased risk for this type of stone.

An acid urine also decreases citrate formation (the natural inhibitor of stones) by the kidneys, making a calcium oxalate stone more likely.

Fat Malabsorption

Bowel disease or diarrhea can cause a problem with fat digestion that affects the interaction of calcium and oxalate in the intestine. (See "The Calcium Controversy" in Chapter 8.)

If you have ever washed your hands in hard water, you know that a residue stays on your hands when you use soap. This residue is actually a combination of calcium and the fatty acids that comprise soap. In the presence of calcium, two fatty acid molecules stick together with one calcium molecule to make the "goo" that is so hard to clean off your hands. We say that the calcium is "soaped out."

A similar process occurs in your intestines. When the bowel does not absorb fat normally, there are many free fatty acids in the upper intestine. The calcium in the upper intestine sticks to the fatty acid molecules and is "soaped out." Since there is less calcium to bind with oxalate in the first part of the intestine, the oxalate travels to the colon, where it is absorbed. Therefore, fat malabsorption leads to an increased net oxalate absorption and, finally, to increased urinary oxalate.

This process occurs in people with Crohn's disease, fast bowel transit diarrhea, intestinal resections, and people who have had bypass surgery for obesity. It is not usually seen in people with ileostomies because the colon has been removed.

Therefore, any bowel disease that causes fat malabsorption causes more oxalate to be absorbed in the large intestine.

You should now understand why *controlling dietary oxalate* is a critical part of stone management for anyone with bowel disease.

Magnesium and Bowel Disease

Magnesium is an inhibitor of the calcium oxalate system. And, like calcium, magnesium can be "soaped out" of the intestine in people with fat malabsorption caused by bowel disease. Therefore, magnesium depletion can become a problem for these people.

There is little evidence that supplementing magnesium in a normal person will reduce the likelihood of stone formation. However, people with bowel disease may benefit from taking magnesium oxide. Since magnesium tends to be a laxative—as in milk of magnesia—giving magnesium supplements to someone with bowel disease can backfire. Magnesium supplements are not recommended without the advice of your physician. (See Chapter 24, "Medications.")

Treatment for Patients with Bowel Disease

If you have a bowel disease, you need to pay particular attention to the oxalate and fat content of your diet. In general, people with stones and intestinal disease need to

• Increase urinary volume
• Increase urinary pH
• Decrease dietary fat and oxalate

Medullary Sponge Kidney (MSK)

MSK is a congenital condition in which the final ducts leading to the collecting system of the kidneys are unusually broad and cause a slow flow of urine. Stones form in the dilated ducts because of the slow flow of urine, like algae forming on a pond.

It is called "sponge" kidney because the ducts have the appearance of a sponge when seen on X ray. (See Figure 5.) The abnormality may affect one or both kidneys, and symptoms include infection and/or stone formation.

Sponge kidney is particularly common in southern Italians, although it is found in all population groups. Frequently, people with MSK have increased calcium excretion and decreased citrate formation.

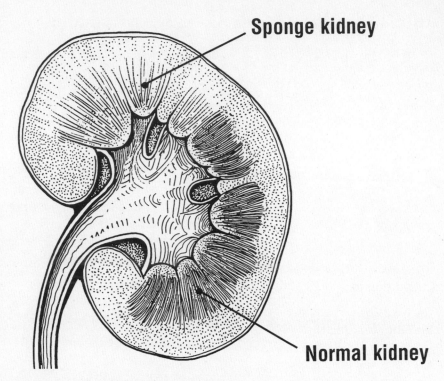

Sponge kidney

Normal kidney

Figure 5.   Medullary Sponge Kidney
The medullary sponge kidney has a "spongy" appearance only on the
intravenous pyelogram (IVP).

Some people with sponge kidney make stones only occasionally.
Others have virulent stone disease and need to be treated with thiazides
and potassium citrate (see Chapter 24), as well as dietary control.

Hyperparathyroidism

There are four (and occasionally five or even six) parathyroid glands
in your neck. They regulate calcium metabolism in your body. When
the amount of calcium in your bloodstream is too low, the glands
make more *parathyroid hormone (PTH)*. When blood calcium is too
high, the glands make less PTH.

It is possible to have benign growths in the parathyroid glands
that cause PTH levels to be inappropriately high. In other words,

PTH can be secreted at a high rate even though blood calcium is high.

When the amount of calcium in your bloodstream stays too high, more calcium spills into the urine and may cause stone formation.

Everyone with stone disease should have blood tests (see "Tests" in Chapter 13) that include a serum (blood) calcium level to determine if *hyperparathyroidism* is contributing to or causing the stone problem.

In most cases when hyperparathyroidism is detected, surgical removal of the abnormal parathyroid gland is warranted. Otherwise, the stone formation will continue.

Milk-Alkali Syndrome and Ulcers

In addition to hyperparathyroidism, milk-alkali syndrome may contribute to kidney stones. This condition occurs when people with ulcer disease take too much antacid and milk to neutralize stomach acid. They may make stones because calcium absorption is markedly increased.

This milk-alkali syndrome has not been as prevalent since the development of drugs such as ranitidine (Zantac) and famotidine (Pepcid) for the treatment of ulcers or stomach acidity. I had a patient who took huge amounts of calcium carbonate antacids and then made numerous apatite stones. (See "Calcium-Containing Stones" in Chapter 4.) His stone-forming problem stopped when we managed his ulcer disease with ranitidine. (See Chapter 24, "Medications.")

Anatomic Abnormalities

There are numerous anatomic abnormalities that can occur in the urinary tract. Some are congenital, others can be acquired through disease or trauma. These anatomic abnormalities encourage stone formation either by slowing the flow of urine, resulting in *reflux* (a backup of urine into the kidney), or by causing voiding problems.

While it is impossible to detail all of the different anatomic problems that affect kidney stone formation, the following are the most common.

Slow Flow of Urine

It takes time for a small crystal to grow into a stone. If crystals sit in one place in the kidney, or adhere to the lining of the urinary tract, stones have time to grow. If the urine flow is fast, the crystals wash out.

People with a *calyceal diverticulum* have a place in the upper urinary tracts where the urine flow is stagnant. (See Figure 6.) People with *ureteropelvic dysproportion* have a "kink" in the ureter where stones can hang up. (See Figure 7.) If medical therapy does not stop the stone disease in these people, surgery may be required to eliminate the anatomic problem.

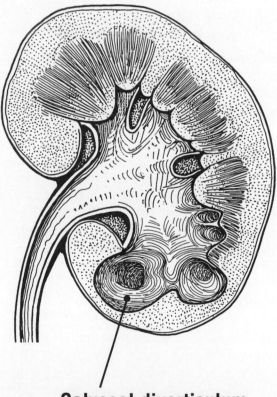

Calyceal diverticulum

Figure 6.   Calyceal Diverticulum
Calyceal diverticula are areas in the kidney that become "blown out" and lose their sharp points.

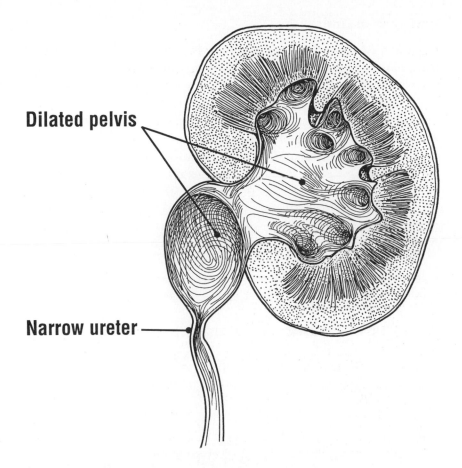

Dilated pelvis

Narrow ureter

Figure 7.   Ureteropelvic Dysproportion
Some people are born with a narrow area in the ureter close to the pelvis of
the kidney. This condition is called ureteropelvic dysproportion.

Reflux of Urine

When urine moves backward from the bladder into the kidney, the
kidney is more prone to infection and to struvite (infection) stones.

One cause of reflux is found in people with two ureters, one
draining the upper pole of the kidney and one the lower pole. Frequently, the upper-pole ureter has an abnormal insertion into the
bladder, allowing urine to reflux into this part of the kidney.

Voiding Problems

Problems with the voiding process may be neurological, such as those that occur with multiple sclerosis, strokes, diabetes, or spinal cord injury. There may also be an obstruction to outflow from the bladder, which is seen in prostate problems, strictures from trauma, venereal disease, or previous catheterization. Problems with voiding make bladder stones more likely.

The most common cause of bladder outflow problems is enlargement of the prostate gland in the older male.

In addition, some older people can develop bladder stones with acquired changes in the end of the spinal column. These include *spinal stenosis,* or narrowing of the spinal canal due to bone changes that occur with aging.

We cannot always change the anatomy, but we can change its consequences through proper diet and treatment.

Paralysis and Immobilization

Whenever the skeleton is not bearing weight, the body begins to remove calcium from the bones. This is one of the chief problems in people with spinal cord injuries.

I have seen several patients who made their first stones after a severe car accident that put them into bed for several months. When these patients are unable to stand and bear weight, the body removes mineral from the skeleton. This results in an increase in urinary calcium that is called *resorptive hypercalciuria,* since it comes from bone resorption.

The problem is further complicated by the fact that bladder function may also be compromised. Frequently, the catheters needed to empty the urinary tract cause an increased incidence of infection. The combination of infection and increased gravel-like material in the urine can be virulent.

To prevent bone resorption, the body must bear weight.

If a paralyzed person is given passive exercise in bed, calcium will still resorb from the bones. However, use of a tilt-table, so that the skeleton must bear weight, slows or stops the process of bone resorption.

Interestingly, bone resorption is one of the anticipated problems of prolonged weightlessness in space travel and has been of considerable concern to NASA. NASA scientists have done extensive studies on how weightlessness might affect stone disease.

Renal Tubular Acidosis (RTA)

RTA is an inherited defect in the kidney's ability to excrete acid and lower the urinary pH to normal levels. (See "Acid and Base" in Chapter 3.) This defect is also associated with a decreased ability to make citrate.

People with RTA, similar to those with an ileostomy or chronic diarrhea, have low urinary citrate, making calcium oxalate stone formation more likely. In addition, people with RTA tend to have excessive calcium excretion.

If the cause of your stone(s) is in doubt, if you are a young woman with a calcium oxalate stone, or if you made stones before age twenty, you should ask your doctor if a test for RTA is appropriate.

Acquired RTA in Glaucoma Patients

Some people with glaucoma form kidney stones while they are on carbonic anhydrase inhibitors (e.g., Diamox or acetazolamide) to lower eye pressure.

Although these drugs lower eye pressure, they can also lower urinary citrate and increase urinary calcium. They create an acquired form of RTA that goes away when the drug is stopped. Patients can take potassium citrate supplements while the acetazolamide is continued in order to minimize the tendency to make stones.

It is often a difficult clinical decision whether or not to continue the carbonic anhydrase inhibitors in a person who has made stones. The risk of stone disease must be weighed against a possible progression of the eye disease.

Cystinuria

Cystinuria is an inherited error of metabolism that causes the kidneys to "leak" cystine. This amino acid is very insoluble and forms into cystine stones. People with cystinuria may also make any of the other stone types.

Although it can occur at any age, this condition is often suspected if a person less than twenty years of age makes stones, particularly when no stone has been available for analysis. These stones also may have a characteristic appearance on an X ray.

People with recurrent stone episodes where no stone is available for analysis should be screened for cystinuria.

People with cystinuria must follow the directives on fluid consumption to the letter. More than any other recommendation in this book, these people need to consume twelve to sixteen glasses of water each day and must have a urinary output over 2500 cc per day.

Oxalosis

Oxalosis is an inherited disease that causes abnormally high oxalate excretions. It occurs in small children and results in calcified kidneys and blood vessels. These children end up on dialysis at an early age.

Some adults have very high oxalate excretions without a good explanation. They appear to have inherited an incomplete form of the disease. This situation should be considered in anyone with an unexpectedly high oxalate excretion. Adults with this condition may benefit from supplements of vitamin B_6, pyridoxine. (See Chapter 24, "Medications.")

If you are suffering from the various special situations discussed in this chapter you will, in all likelihood, be under the constant supervision of a physician. While the dietary guidelines in this book have been tested and are safe for all of the situations described, you should review any and all dietary changes with your personal physician.

10

DIETING YOUR WAY TO A KIDNEY STONE

My weight goes up and down. I've literally lost a thousand pounds. The first stone came after I was on a liquid diet for four months.

You know how you read little articles about home remedies . . . and one that's been around for a long time is drinking vinegar. It's good for arthritis and just clears away the viruses. So I mixed the vinegar with grape juice and apple juice and drank it every morning. It felt wonderful to drink it. And I would have a huge bowl of fresh strawberries or raspberries along with this drink. I thought I couldn't be healthier. I guess that's what set off this last kidney stone.

It seems that there is always a new diet or health fad on the market. The purpose of most diets is to get rid of excess, undesirable fat. There are also supplements people take to prevent colds, alleviate arthritis, cure baldness, or improve their sex lives. All of these have the potential to lead to the formation of kidney stones.

The Problem with Rapid Weight Loss

Quick weight-loss diets cause an increased turnover of your body tissue. You are "burning off" body weight stored in your system, which represents an infusion of the same substances in your system

69

as the digestion of meat. (See "Protein and Kidney Stones" in Chapter 8.)

As the excess tissue breaks down, your kidney is presented with the same basic waste products that you generate when you eat a large meat meal. These products include uric acid, oxalates, and other acids. In other words, the kidney has the same job to do whether you are metabolizing your own excess tissue or a large steak. Rapid weight loss is as bad as, or potentially worse than, overeating protein when it comes to causing stone disease.

Ketosis

Rapid weight loss produces a condition called *ketosis,* which is particularly bad for stone formers.

When the body begins to break down stored fat for energy, the blood levels of two organic acids increase. The accumulation of these substances is called ketosis because the substances contain a chemical group called a "ketone." The accumulation of these organic acids makes the pH of the urine acid all of the time. An acid urine is ideal for stone formation.

When weight loss is slow and gradual, the levels of the two ketones is never very high, so the effect on urinary chemistry is small. However, crash diets allow significant amounts of the ketones to pile up in the bloodstream and spill into the urine. This is why we frequently give potassium bicarbonate citrate supplements to stone formers who are beginning a diet. The administration of base tends to raise the urinary pH, making stone formation less likely. (See "Acid and Base" in Chapter 3.)

Stone formers should be extremely cautious about crash dieting and should certainly consult a physician before using bicarbonate supplements in conjunction with a diet.

Fad Dieting

Fad diets are never-ending. While some are balanced and sensible, many that catch on with the public promise quick results with little effort. These are the ones that lead to nutritional deficiencies and stress the kidneys.

Liquid Protein Diets

Liquid protein diets have been in and out of vogue for the past decade. In the early 1980s, an extraordinary number of people who were referred to me were taking liquid protein. My secretary began to kid me by saying that she could give the patients the same advice that I gave them—namely, to stop this type of dieting—and they would not have to see me.

One of the classic profiles of a stone former describes the overeater who needs to lose weight as well as lower intake of animal protein. We do not want that person to take off 25 pounds in a month on a liquid protein diet and form stones.

Liquid formula diets are found in the supermarket and in pharmacies. The dieter experiences quick weight loss, which taxes the kidneys and urine output. Other drawbacks to liquid protein diets are a dependence on a particular brand or product, an inability to readjust to healthy eating habits, and, finally, rebound weight gain.

Liquid protein diets increase urinary uric acid and make urinary pH more acid. They are great for my business, not for your kidneys.

Low-Carbohydrate, High-Fat Diets

Diets that emphasize protein and limit carbohydrates are particularly bad for the stone former. They produce ketosis and an initial rapid weight loss from water depletion.

I strongly recommend against this type of diet for anyone who has made stones.

High-Carbohydrate, Low-Fat Diets

These diets restrict fat to 10 percent of total calories, with carbohydrate levels at 80 percent. The diet produces rapid weight loss and is nutritionally adequate. Stone formers, however, must be sure that the carbohydrates in the diet are not from food sources high in oxalates.

Any rapid weight-loss program can predispose you to stone formation. However, this form of diet is theoretically not as bad as others. In our experience, high-carbohydrate dieting does not seem to produce stones as virulently as, for example, the high-fat, low-carbohydrate diets.

Other Weight-Loss Programs

Various programs offer diets that are well balanced but associated with the problems of rapid weight loss. Some of these diet programs provide reduced-calorie diets in a prepackaged form. These may be appealing, but they may include high-oxalate foods (like spinach) that can sabotage your efforts.

Very Low-Calorie Diets

Very low-calorie diets of fewer than 800 calories are reserved for the morbidly obese for whom other diet programs have failed. Typically, these diets are high in protein, in the form of milk or egg protein, with the remaining food choices in carbohydrates with very little fat. These diets promote rapid weight loss due to sodium and water loss. They can also lead to ketosis and an increase in uric acid in the blood. This raises the potential for gout as well as uric acid stones.

Finally, the inability of most rapid dieters to maintain their lowered weights makes this type of diet, at best, risky.

The best approach for the overweight stone former is to learn once and for all what food choices are necessary for permanent change.

Fad Health Regimens

Take morning and evening a teaspoon of onions, calcined in a fire-shovel into white ashes, in white wine. An ounce will often dissolve the stone.
—CLARENCE MEYER, *AMERICAN FOLK MEDICINE*

Today's health-conscious consumer will often go to dangerous extremes in an effort to stay healthy or cure a chronic health problem. While I am confident that my patients will not resort to onion ash in white wine, many come to me with stone disease brought on by so-called health regimens.

Megadoses of Vitamin C

My mother and girlfriend had convinced me of the virtues of vitamin C even though I kept saying: "I don't believe in this." I was taking over 2000 milligrams a day trying to ward off the cold season right before the first (stone) episode.

Vitamin C can be converted to oxalate, a component of the majority of kidney stones. It is not clear whether small amounts of vitamin C supplements—250 milligrams to 500 milligrams a day—will actually increase urinary oxalate. Larger amounts may, but data on this point are controversial.

The effect of vitamin C on urinary oxalate differs from one person to another. While there have been studies that suggest that small amounts of vitamin C do not raise the average amount of oxalate excreted, I have seen patients in whom vitamin C supplements unequivocally raised urinary oxalate.

Furthermore, vitamin C is an acid (ascorbic acid) and tends to lower urinary pH. The lower urinary pH will lower urinary citrate, a natural inhibitor of kidney stones. (See Chapter 8 for vitamin C recommendations.)

Eating Disorders

Eating disorders are frequently associated with kidney stone formation. It doesn't matter what type of eating disorder a person has—bulimia, anorexia, or compulsive eating—they can all lead to the formation of kidney stones because they throw off the chemical balance in the body.

For example, people with *bulimia* alternate between stuffing themselves with food and then fasting or vomiting. Calcium and oxalate excretions rise dramatically during a stuff and fall dramatically during the fasting.

I had a patient who admitted to a severe eating disorder who consented to let me measure her urinary chemistries during a stuff and fast. (She had weight swings of 30 to 40 pounds in a two- to three-month period.)

Fast: Calcium—90 mg; Oxalate—16 mg; Citrate—480 mg
Stuff: Calcium—600 mg; Oxalate—56 mg; Citrate—195 mg

The calcium oxalate product increased with the stuff more than twenty-five times, and the inhibitory action of citrate was reduced to less than half. This patient is over fifty times more likely to make stones during her stuffs.

Many people who are obsessed with thinness have additional habits that predispose them to kidney stones. I had one such patient who smoked two packs of cigarettes and took eight laxatives a day. (See "Laxative Abuse," following.) She also took *analgesics* regularly. She made dozens of stones.

The first obstacle in treating any person with an eating disorder is to help that person recognize and overcome it. Kidney stones may be the least part of the problem. Extreme dieting or overeating can lead to many serious medical problems. Some of these have the potential to be life threatening.

Laxative Abuse

Some people develop a habit of overusing laxatives or enemas. The overuse of laxatives is almost always a female problem. The psychological reasons for this habit are beyond the scope of this book. The consequences, however, can be a peculiar form of stone formation that is similar to the kind of stone problem sometimes seen in children with chronic dysentery in underdeveloped countries.

The biochemical result of laxative abuse is chronic *acidosis* because of the continuing loss of bicarbonate in the stool. The urinary pH remains acid all of the time. (See "Acid and Base" in Chapter 3.) Indeed, many of these women have a systemic acidosis that also leads to loss of mineral from the skeleton and osteoporosis.

The use of laxatives also causes a loss of potassium. The potassium depletion causes the kidney to make an unusually large amount of *ammonium* to compensate, and this causes a rare type of stone called *ammonium acid urate* (AAU). This is a stone we virtually never see except in patients with some kind of unusual bowel problem.

Most of the women who make AAU-containing stones are quite thin, even anorectic. They are borderline malnourished. It is not surprising that their stones are the same in composition as those seen in children in underdeveloped countries who are malnourished or who have chronic dysentery. These patients have acquired a form of bowel disease that predisposes them to making both uric acid and calcium oxalate stones as well as the rare AAU stone.

The most important point with these patients is to recognize and acknowledge the condition, and then find ways of creating more normal bowel habits.

Some people sporadically purge themselves with various formulations such as grape juice and vinegar. These habits may also be the cause of kidney stones.

How Stone Formers Should Diet

If you need to lose weight, by all means do so. However, you should recognize that the process of weight loss, and its simultaneous water depletion, increases your chance of making stones—particularly if the weight loss is rapid.

The best way to lose weight is to combine a nutritionally balanced diet with exercise and behavior modifications. These guidelines apply to the stone former as well as the general population. A balanced diet makes ketosis less likely. Increasing your fluid intake while dieting also helps to minimize the likelihood of stone formation.

Sometimes, when we have a person who has made stones and needs to lose weight, we will give potassium citrate supplements during the period of dieting to provide some protection against stone formation.

Finally, do not embark on a "health" regimen without consulting your physician. You may be dieting your way to a kidney stone.

11

MEN AND STONES

I think that passing a stone is the male equivalent of giving birth. The pain is so intense, you think you're going to die.

Stone disease is much more common in men than in women. The ratio, however, of male to female stone formers varies widely in populations depending on diet and other factors.

Why Men Make More Kidney Stones

Men generally have a larger muscle mass than women. Hence they have more of the daily breakdown and rebuilding of tissue that results in metabolic waste. And an increase in metabolic waste predisposes people to stone formation.

Men generally eat more meat than women do. In the United States, males over the age of twenty consume a daily average of 90 grams of protein whereas women, on average, consume only 65 grams. However, when we compile dietary histories of stone formers, we often find protein intakes much higher than these levels. It is not rare to find a male stone former in his forties consuming over 200 grams of protein on many days. (See Chapter 8.)

The male urinary tract is more complicated than the female urinary tract. (See Figure 1, page 11.) The male urethra has two additional portions and it is here that problems can occur. The upper portion, the prostatic urethra, passes through the prostate gland. The lower portion, the penile urethra, runs along the lower part of the penis.

The Prostate Gland

The complexity of the male urinary tract is further complicated by the position of the prostate gland. The function of the prostate gland is to package sperm into a protective fluid for ejaculation. Any enlargement of the prostate gland can potentially impinge on the free flow of urine through this part of the urethra. As men get older, the prostate gland continually enlarges. The urinary stream becomes less forceful. No sixty-year-old man has a stream as strong as he had at forty, nor does a forty-year-old man have the stream he had at twenty.

In most cases, the decrease in urinary force is inconsequential. However, in some men, the prostate gland becomes enlarged enough to put pressure on the urethra, causing the condition known as *BPH* (*benign prostatic hypertrophy*). BPH makes it difficult to empty the bladder completely, so that some urine remains in the bladder at all times. Men with BPH have

- Difficulty initiating voiding
- Weakness of stream (they need to be close to the toilet to avoid accidents)
- Stream dribbling (a sensation of needing to urinate frequently with small amounts of urine coming out each time)
- Frequent nighttime urination because they are unable to empty the bladder totally

There is nothing inherently dangerous about BPH. It is not prostate cancer but a normal aging process that makes emptying the bladder more difficult. The *detrussor muscle*, which causes the bladder to contract and expel urine, can maintain a contraction only for a limited period of time. This may not be long enough for someone with BPH to empty the bladder.

I encourage men with prostate problems to spend a few moments "re-peeing." This involves urinating, stopping, counting to thirty, and urinating again. It may then be possible to empty the bladder more completely.

Stricture of the Penile Urethra

Occasionally we see men with a narrowing of the penile urethra. This situation can occur as a result of a gonorrhea infection, catheterization, or penile trauma such as a zipper injury.

Both BPH and urethral stricture minimize bladder outflow. Anatomically, the urethra is larger than the ureter, so most stones that reach the bladder usually pass easily from that point. However, when the bladder outflow is obstructed, crystals and small stones may accumulate in the bladder. Furthermore, when the bladder has been operating under increased pressure, little pouches, or diverticula, may develop in the wall. Stones can accumulate in these diverticula. (See Figure 8.)

Therefore, almost all bladder stones occur in men. Females with bladder stones almost always have some problem with the neurological function of the bladder muscle that contracts and expels urine.

Prostatitis

Prostatitis is an inflammation of the prostate gland causing acute symptoms such as an urgency to urinate, frequent need to urinate, and a very weak stream. This condition can occur both with and

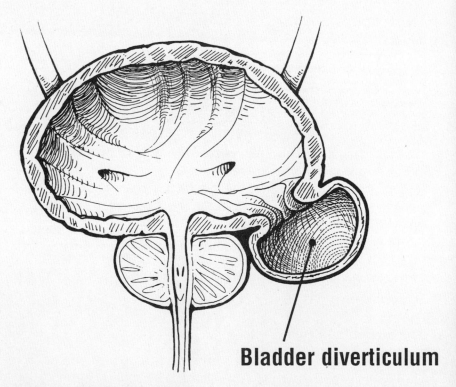

Bladder diverticulum

Figure 8.   Bladder Diverticulum
Bladder diverticula frequently form in men who have prostate problems.

without infection. When there is fever or chills, a bacterial infection is almost always present. Whether or not there is an infection, the presence of constant prostate symptoms should receive prompt attention, because they are easier and more successfully treated before they are allowed to progress.

Since this is not a book about prostatitis, I will only discuss the role this inflammation plays in the person with stone disease.

If a man suffers from prostatitis, he has difficulty emptying his bladder, so the crystals that form kidney stones are more likely to accumulate there. Many men are annoyed by having to make frequent trips to the bathroom, so they instinctively reduce fluid intake. This is exactly what you do not want to do because it makes stone formation more likely. (See Chapter 7.) Moreover, if there are recurring prostate infections in the presence of stone disease, the possibility of infecting a stone is increased.

Prostatitis is not a venereal disease. It is not a condition that the male catches from the female nor, under ordinary conditions, can the male give the female anything. However, since certain venereal diseases such as *chlamydia* can be confused with ordinary prostatitis, it is wise to consult a physician.

Prostatitis is sometimes brought on by a sudden decrease in sexual activity. I treated an unusually severe case of prostatitis in a man whose wife was a nurse called to Iraq during Desert Storm. He was left with a sudden decrease in the frequency with which he ejaculated. Except when there is fever, ejaculation often helps prostatitis.

Alcohol and Prostatitis

Alcohol may make any prostate problem worse. A large amount of alcohol makes the detrussor muscle, which causes the bladder to contract and expel urine, contract less efficiently. Urine is then left in the bladder, which acts like a petri dish on which more bacteria can grow, in turn aggravating the prostatic symptoms.

While small amounts of alcohol probably make no difference, we recommend that men with prostatitis not drink heavily.

Pain Patterns

Pain patterns are different in men and women, particularly for stones in the upper parts of the ureter and the kidney. As discussed in

Chapter 6, the ducts that drain the testicle and the upper part of the ureter have a similar embryological origin. Hence, a man will frequently feel pain in the testicle from a stone in the kidney on the same side. Many men with kidney stones are misdiagnosed as having epididymitis, an inflammation of the testicle. (See Chapter 6, "Why Kidney Stones Are So Painful.")

12

WOMEN AND STONES

"You cannot tell the he from she."
　　　　　　　　　—ROLAND YOUNG, 1887–1953

The classic ratio for kidney stone formation has been 5 to1, male to female. Increasingly, kidney stones are becoming an equal opportunity condition. The changing ratio of male to female stone formers may be due to a greater similarity in what men and women eat. There are specific data from Sweden where the male/female ratio is almost even; this correlates with a diet rich in animal protein for both sexes. There are also a number of situations in which women are *more* likely to form stones.

Why Women Make Kidney Stones

Many women have a lower urinary flow, which increases the relative frequency of stone formation. Whether this aversion to drinking fluids is influenced by social attitudes toward ladylike behavior and bathroom habits, the use of public toilets, or any number of other reasons, there are many women who just do not take in enough fluids. Low urinary volume is a very common problem in female stone formers, more so than in men.

Women are more prone to urinary tract infections. For this reason, kidney stone disease has a greater potential to create severe clinical problems in women. A minor stone problem can easily become a major one if it becomes complicated by infection.

One of the more common times women form stones is in the latter part of a pregnancy. I have seen close to a hundred stone episodes in pregnant women, and all but two were in the last trimester.

Women are more likely to take large amounts of analgesics for menstrual cramps and headaches. Taken in large quantities over long periods of time, these medications, such as *NSAIDS* (nonsteroidal, anti-inflammatory drugs such as ibuprofen and naproxen) and acetaminophen, can cause damage to the *papillae* of the kidney. Injured papillae can seed a stone as well as complicate the stone-forming process.

I saw one patient from South America who was taking large amounts of an NSAID for her menstrual pains. One doctor was actually injecting her with *Butazolidin* (an anti-inflammatory) on a monthly basis. Her many episodes of colic were not even stones. They were caused by sloughed pieces of her kidney damaged by excessive NSAIDS.

Fluids

Many of my female patients have psychological barriers regarding urination. And their decision to restrict fluids is often unconscious.

One woman who had been in the Israeli army found the need to urinate without privacy particularly disturbing. Surrounded by soldiers of both sexes, she deliberately avoided fluids and sometimes urinated only once a day. Obviously, part of treating her stone problem was deconditioning her military experience.

Women who travel a lot, like all travelers, may avoid fluids. My female patients seem to have more ski-induced stone disease than do the men. One patient of mine made all of her stones when she was skiing in Colorado. As we will discuss in Chapter 16, "Lifestyles of the Kidney Stone Former," high-altitude living predisposes you to stone formation by facilitating dehydration through the skin. In addition, women often describe the difficulty of taking off cumbersome ski clothing in order to urinate.

Whether or not urination is an indelicate subject, it is important to address fluid intake. In many instances, it is the only therapeutic recommendation needed for some female stone formers. Incidentally, it is also one of the most important aspects of treating urinary tract infections in women.

Urinary Tract Infections

There are many women who develop urinary tract infections simply because they don't drink enough fluids. One of the hardest things in stone management is to uncondition that behavior.

If a urinary tract with a tiny retained stone becomes infected, there is the danger that the infection will be extremely difficult to eradicate. For example, an infection associated with a splinter in your finger is rarely eliminated until the splinter is removed.

If the infection happens to be with an organism like *Proteus*, then the infection itself may generate its own kind of stone material, *struvite*. (See "Struvite Stones" in Chapter 4.) This is how dangerous stones begin, and they can ultimately destroy kidneys.

There is cause for concern when a woman with a retained stone develops a urinary tract infection. Follow-up cultures to be sure that the urine is sterile and infection-free are always necessary when a woman with a retained stone is treated for a urinary infection.

Pregnancy

The pregnant woman has to provide enough calcium in her blood to form a whole new skeleton, and that calcium has to come from somewhere. Since 98 percent of the calcium in the human body is in the bones, if all of the calcium for the fetal skeleton came from the mother's body, she would pay a very expensive price. There is actually an old saw that predicts losing "a tooth a child," referring to what was probably a common occurrence before the modern understanding of calcium depletion.

In order to protect the mother's skeleton (and teeth), there are profound alterations in the calcium metabolism of a pregnant woman. In very simple terms, more calcium is absorbed from the intestine. If there is not enough, some is taken from the bones. Particularly in the latter months of pregnancy, the mother's skeleton will lose bone if she is not taking enough calcium. As more calcium is absorbed from the upper intestine, more oxalate is available in the lower intestine. (See "The Calcium Controversy" in Chapter 8.)

Nature provides protection, though, against the potential adverse effects of higher urinary calcium and oxalate, which predispose to stone formation. The pregnant woman makes more citrate and other natural inhibitors of kidney stones. The levels of these inhibitors can be several times those of a nonpregnant woman. If they were not present, most women would make stones in the eighth and ninth months of a pregnancy.

Another factor that makes the pregnant woman more likely to create stones is her diminished bladder capacity. As the fetus grows, there is less room in the pelvis for a full bladder. Therefore, to minimize the constant trips to the bathroom, many women deliberately avoid fluids toward the end of a pregnancy. Since urinary calcium is at its highest levels in the last trimester, this low urine flow can result in stone formation.

I treated one pregnant woman who had formed multiple stones. She commuted one and a half hours to work in New York City. Because of the commute, she felt she could not drink as much fluid as I recommended. Therefore, I had to give her a choice: For the last month and a half of her pregnancy she had to either stop working or move in with her mother who lived in Manhattan. She decided to move into Manhattan, where her commute was only fifteen minutes, for the last part of her pregnancy. (She avoided another stone episode.)

When I have to manage a woman who has made stones and who decides to become pregnant, I do not usually restrict her calcium intake because that could compromise the fetus or leech too much calcium from her bones. I do place her on a low-oxalate diet and encourage her to take enough fluids to make 2 liters of urine a day. She may have to stay close to a bathroom and restrict her activities to enable her to accomplish this goal during the last trimester, but that inconvenience may be the only way to allow her to complete a pregnancy safely.

I may also supplement her with potassium citrate and recommend that her calcium supplements for the pregnancy be given as calcium citrate. (See Chapter 24, "Medications.")

Since the stakes are so high, I cannot recommend strongly enough that a woman who has made a stone and who is carrying a baby seek expert advice beyond what is in this chapter. Any pregnant woman should discuss a prior stone problem with a knowledgeable physician prior to taking any supplements, even over-the-counter products.

When a woman makes stones, particularly before age thirty, we suspect the case is not routine. The woman may have an eating disorder such as bulimia (see Chapter 10). Occasionally, we find renal tubular acidosis (RTA), or a vitamin fad (see Chapter 8). She may have cystinuria. There may be a family incidence of stone disease and early osteoporosis.

Although the incidence of stone formation in women is not as yet equal to that in men, certain factors put women at special risk for stone disease. Recognizing these factors, increasing fluids, and eliminating problem substances and habits can change the outcome.

13

THE WORKUP

*Is there any way to tell the age of a stone? Like, it's a
year, it just started walking.*

*I probably don't see the doctor as often as I should. I
don't want to hear the bad news.*

Everyone's stone problem is different. Some people have experienced
a single stone, whereas others have had multiple surgical procedures
for stone disease and may have been threatened with the loss of a
kidney. It is necessary to place these two extremes in perspective
because it is not practical or cost effective to do an A-to-Z workup
on everyone.

How, then, do I rate the severity of your stone disease? And, more
importantly, how do I decide the level of intervention and compli-
ance that is necessary to prevent a recurrence?

Risk Assessment

The first part of the workup is a risk assessment to determine the
severity of your problem. The number of tests that will be run, as
well as the procedures, medications, and dietary advice you will
receive, must make sense for your specific situation.

Essentially, your risk potential will fall in one of three general
categories:

- *At high risk* for recurrence as well as potential complications
- *At risk* for further stone formation
- *At low risk/probability* of forming another stone

86

Those at highest risk will have more intense workups and treatments.

The Workup

There are seven parts to the medical workup. Each contributes to the physician's understanding of how complicated your problem is and how aggressive your treatment must be. The following is a breakdown of each aspect of the workup in order to explain where it is appropriate and why it is included. Not everyone receives the same workup.

Please note: The information in this chapter is not meant for self-diagnosis or as a substitute for a medical workup. Nothing here should replace the considered opinion of a knowledgeable physician. It is up to your doctor to determine the necessary history, tests, and follow-up that you will require.

Family History

Genetics play a large role in stone disease. A family history may uncover other family members with kidney stones or other conditions (e.g., chronic gastric problems) that may predispose you to stones.

Underlying Medical Conditions

The physician must look for hyperparathyroidism, RTA, cystinuria, and any other medical conditions such as bowel disease, gout, or paralysis that might predispose you to continued kidney stone formation. As mentioned in Chapter 9 (under "Acquired RTA in Glaucoma Patients"), different prescription drugs may increase calcium excretion or otherwise cause the formation of stones. Your physician should also check for bone disease or evidence of infection.

The combination of stones plus infection can be particularly dangerous. (See "Struvite Stones" in Chapter 4 and "Urinary Tract Infection" in Chapter 12.) Stone formers with infections must go to great lengths to try to avoid the recurrence of such a situation. This means not only trying to prevent urinary infections but also preventing any type of stone from forming. Strict fluid and dietary regimens would be required, as well as medication.

Urinary Tract Abnormalities

Anatomic abnormalities lead to a number of special situations that must be determined and individually treated. (See "Anatomical Abnormalities" in Chapter 9.)

Dietary Aberrations

If I can determine the cause of your stones from a fad diet or vitamin supplement program, I will be less inclined to do an elaborate workup. (See "Fad Dieting" in Chapter 10.)

I saw a patient who had purchased a tomato farm in New Jersey. In September, after his first full season of farming, he made his first stone. While small amounts of tomatoes are probably inconsequential, he had been "nibbling" on tomatoes all day for several months. The sudden increase in oxalates caused him to make a stone. When I know why someone makes stones, I can recommend a dietary prescription without putting that person through multiple tests.

I also look for other dietary aberrations such as a low fluid intake, or a high calcium, oxalate, sodium, or protein consumption. If I feel that an eating disorder is underlying the stone formation, I try to get the person to understand and deal with that issue.

Personal History

I look for unusual histories that may have caused the stone, such as people who travel extensively and cannot access water, or people who live in the desert and might be prone to dehydration. They are all at an increased risk of stone formation. Then there are jobs where people consciously restrict liquid to avoid urinating all day, or occupations that can result in severe dehydration, such as that of a lifeguard or pizza parlor worker. (Working next to a hot oven all day may generate a large fluid loss through the skin.) People with a history of major weight swings may have dieted their way to a stone. (See Chapter 10.)

Stone History

I need to know the precise details of your previous stone episodes. If you can provide accurate data, I can plan a more appropriate approach to your problem.

• *How many stones have you passed?*   Someone with multiple stones is much more likely to have another stone. If there have
been multiple stones in a given family, I may want to work up at least
one member of the family extensively. This may tell me a lot about
the others in the family.

• *Is there an underlying medical condition that makes it more
likely you will make more stones?*   A person with sponge kidney
who has already made four stones has a high probability of making
more. Or, if someone has a stone before the age of twenty, there is
an extremely high possibility that they have some metabolic disorder
causing it.

• *Was the stone difficult or "easy" to pass?*   While passing
a stone "easily" is not a happy experience, it is better than requiring
urological intervention. I will be much more aggressive in
evaluating someone who had to be instrumented by the urologist
to assist passage of a stone (see Chapter 25, "Technology") than
with someone who did not have that much trouble. That might be
relevant if somebody asks me, "Can I fly an airplane?" or "Can I
travel?"

• *What type of stone is it?*   The type of stone(s) you have will
determine the diet and medication that will be recommended. While
it is possible to make an assessment of the probable type of mineral
in a stone from the X ray or eating history, the stone analysis is an
important clue for the doctor.

• *Is there metabolic or surgical activity?*   "Surgical activity"
is when a stone is producing symptoms or is being passed or causing
obstruction. "Metabolic activity" means that new stones are forming
or existing ones are growing bigger, and nothing is moving or causing a blockage.

The distinction between metabolic and surgical activity is important. Suppose a person comes to me having passed five stones. One
had to be removed with a cystoscopic procedure. (See Chapter 25,
"Technology.") His X rays show two retained stones in the right kidney and none in the left. We institute dietary and lifestyle changes
that we hope will be enough to stop further stone formation. Four
months later he passes a stone on the right side. Has our prevention
regimen failed?

A new X ray shows only one stone remaining in the right kidney.
The size of the stone he passed corresponds to that of the stone which
is no longer visible in the right kidney. This patient has not made new

stones. He has surgical activity because he suffered pain and passed a stone. However, he has no metabolic activity. He has not made a new stone; he passed a pre-existing one. There is no need to change our prevention regimen.

On the other hand, suppose the same patient passes no stones after his initial visit with me. Six months later, I order an X ray that now shows the two stones in the right kidney are bigger, and a small stone is now visible in the left kidney. Even though the patient has had no symptoms and no clinical problems with his stones, there is metabolic activity. There are more stones forming and evidence that existing stones are growing. I would conclude that the type of diet and lifestyle changes we have tried are insufficient to control the stone formation and that additional medication is probably in order.

This is metabolic activity without surgical activity, and it indicates that a change in diet, habits, and/or medication is warranted.

• *Do you have retained stones, and did you need to have a stone removed surgically or with instruments*? It is important to determine whether your stones have recently grown and whether they are continuing to grow. Let us say that I am following a patient with two small stones, and the patient has an episode of colic. When a kidney X ray shows that there is only one 2-millimeter stone left, I am happy that one existing stone has passed. If, six months later, I get a film and there are now three stones and they are not 2 millimeters but 4 millimeters, I know that my treatment is failing and I have to step up the intensity of the program.

• *Did you have procedures in the past?* Someone who has had three or four stones and had *extracorporeal shock wave lithotripsy* (ESWL, see Chapter 25), or someone who has had multiple treatments for urinary obstruction, has four retained stones in one kidney and two in the other, will need an extensive workup. That person's dietary and treatment regimen will be demanding.

• *What is the size of the stone?* A typical 2-millimeter stone will eventually come out on its own if you take enough fluids. On the other hand, a larger 10-millimeter stone usually does not pass by itself. Some kind of urological intervention is usually needed.

Most people pass a stone spontaneously. I will be more aggressive in evaluating the cause of stone disease in someone with larger stones that have required a urological procedure.

Tests

There are a number of basic tests that a stone former is likely to encounter. These tests help to rule out or confirm underlying physical causes of the stone. Not everyone is given the full range of tests, as they are not necessary for every type of stone. Some tests are fairly expensive and only undertaken when medically necessary. Following is an explanation of the basic screening tests for kidney stones. You may wish to discuss them further with your own physician.

    X rays and sonography
    Stone analysis
    Blood analysis
    Urinalysis and urine chemistries

X rays and Sonography.   Physicians evaluate your urinary tract with X ray and sonography. This helps determine the number, size, and placement of a stone as well as its type. Some stones cast a shadow on an X ray, others do not.

Radiopaque stones cast a shadow. Calcium-containing stones are radiopaque and can be seen on X-ray film. *Radiolucent* stones do not block the X ray and, therefore, do not cast an image. Uric acid stones are radiolucent and cannot be seen by plain X ray. A mixed calcium oxalate–uric acid stone often appears mottled, as parts of it block an X-ray beam and other parts do not.

The *KUB film (kidney, ureter, bladder)* is a simple X-ray view of your abdomen that will show the presence of anything that blocks X rays. While the KUB film may be affected by obesity or too much gas in the large intestine, it can reveal any radiopaque stones. The amount of radiation involved in a KUB film is small.

The *IVP (intravenous pyelogram)* begins with a KUB film. Then an iodine-containing dye is injected into a vein. This dye is concentrated by the kidney in the ureter and the bladder. The dye is radiopaque, so these structures are delineated on the X-ray pictures. If there is any obstruction to the flow of the iodinated material, the location of the obstruction can be seen. Any abnormal anatomy, such as two rather than one ureter coming from a kidney, can also be seen.

The sonogram uses sound waves rather than X rays to image your kidneys. The human ear can hear the sound of frequencies up to about

10,000 cycles per second (cps). The sound waves used in sonography are well over 1 million cps. You cannot hear them. Much as a submarine uses sonar to navigate under water, the sonogram records echoes from your kidneys.

The sonogram can ascertain if the kidneys are obstructed. Often it cannot tell where the kidney is obstructed, only that there is some blockage. It also can detect the presence of stones and will show both calcified radiopaque stones and noncalcified radiolucent stones. However, it cannot detect very small stones as easily as an X ray.

The KUB film is better for small stones as long as the stones have calcium and can be seen on X ray. The sonogram, though, gives no radiation.

The choice of which of these three tests to do depends on the clinical problem that is present and is up to the judgment of your doctor.

Stone Analysis. The appearance of the stone on the various imaging studies outlined above gives clues as to its composition. For example, struvite stones shape themselves to the collecting ducts of the kidney and have "horns" like the antlers of a deer. (See Chapter 4.) However, a precise analysis is invaluable.

Some hospital laboratories use a chemical kit and can generate partial information. Specialty labs use other tests, including x-ray diffraction, and can give much better information.

Whenever possible, stones should be sent to a specialty laboratory. These labs can detail trace minerals that may lead to the origin of the stone, as well as the predominant mineral present. For example, as discussed in Chapter 9, the presence of carbonate apatite mixed with calcium oxalate signals the likelihood of renal tubular acidosis or hyperparathyroidism. Ammonium acid urate indicates an intestinal problem.

Do not be afraid to ask where your stone is going to be analyzed. There is no going back if the analysis is not done right the first time. I know of a patient who carried his stone around in his pocket because he "wanted to keep it." If you have similar thoughts, I would recommend sending your stone for analysis and purchasing one of the "pet rocks" sold in novelty stores instead.

Blood Analysis. Routine blood tests can measure your general health and indicate elevated levels of specific minerals:

- *Calcium.*   Tested to pick up systemic disorders of calcium metabolism. The most important one to identify is hyperparathyroidism.
- *Phosphate.*   If this is low, it suggests hyperparathyroidism or some disorder of renal function. Some people with low serum phosphate may benefit from oral supplements of phosphate.
- *Creatinine.*   The best overall measure of total kidney function.
- *Electrolytes.*   (Sodium, Potassium, Chloride, CO_2). These may give a clue to the presence of renal tubular acidosis or some other systemic metabolic disorder. You may have unrecognized diarrhea or other causes for low potassium that may interact with your stone disease.
- *Uric Acid.*   This substance is the chief component of some stones. It is measured to make sure you do not have a systemic disorder of uric acid metabolism.
- *Sugar.*   To eliminate the possibility of diabetes.
- *Alkaline Phosphatase.*   This enzyme is found in both liver and bone. If an elevated alkaline phosphatase comes from bone, it has important implications for calcium metabolism and underlying bone disease.
- *Cholesterol and Triglycerides.*   The main concern of these tests is kidney stones, but it is important to consider your overall diet. While following a diet to prevent your stones, you should not have to worry about the risk of a heart attack. Moreover, controlling your fat intake is important for weight control. In fact, excess fat ingestion may predispose you to overabsorption of oxalate. (See "Fat Malabsorption" in Chapter 9.)

Urinalysis.   Everyone should be given a routine urinalysis. This test looks to see if the urine contains microscopic crystals. If you are passing crystals, it is fairly certain that the stone-forming process is active. If there is a suggestion of infection, a culture is done.

- *Urine pH Profile.*   Urinary pH provides many clues about the basis of a person's stones. (See "Acid and Base" in Chapter 3.) It screens for the unlikely possibility that you have an inherited disorder of acid formation. It also gives information about your diet and whether you can be a uric acid stone former.

For a urine pH profile, you use a narrow-range pH paper and dip it in freshly voided urine every time you void for three days. There should be at least twenty readings. (If there are not twenty, you are not drinking enough fluids.) Saturate the paper with urine by either urinating into a cup and then dipping the strip into it, or simply urinating across a strip and washing your hands afterward.

* *Cystinuria Screening.*   Anyone with a likely diagnosis of cystinuria should be screened for this disorder. The screening can be done on a single voided urinary specimen. Such a test is usually done when several stones have been passed but not analyzed, or when there is a family history of stones.

* *Twenty-four-Hour Urine Collection.*   Many people are asked to collect one or more twenty-four-hour urine specimens. The collection must be done correctly if the results are to be of any help to your physician.

How to Do a Twenty-four-Hour Urine Collection

If collection is to start at 8 A.M. on Day 1, at 8 A.M. you urinate *into the toilet,* making sure to empty your bladder completely.

Put every drop of urine you make on Day 1 into a container, including the first voiding on Day 2, the following morning.

Don't make the mistake of putting the first urine of Day 1 into the collection. That makes the collection more than a day's urine. Do not forget to collect any specimens.

Twenty-four-hour collections should be done as a basis for comparison during treatment. This allows your physician to compare elements in the urine against a baseline to determine if the recommended program is working.

The twenty-four-hour urines that are collected in the hospital at the time a patient is passing a stone are not an indication of the way a patient eats normally. It is possible for a physician to miss the problem when measuring this nonrepresentative urinary chemistry. If you do a twenty-four-hour urine collection from Monday to Tuesday morning, and on Tuesday you eat a large steak, spinach quiche, and have pecan pie for dessert, the urinary chemistries will not reflect the problem.

A twenty-four-hour urine collection measures other elements in the urine:

* *Creatinine.*   This indicates if the collection of urine is appropri-

ate. Creatinine is a by-product of muscle metabolism. The amount produced each day by the body is relatively constant. If the amount of creatinine in the urine does not correspond to the appropriate amount for a person's size and build, the collection was done incorrectly. An inappropriately high level of creatinine means that too much urine has been collected or for too long a period of time. Likewise, a low level means that some specimens have been forgotten.

- *Calcium.*   Abnormally large amounts of calcium give us a clue as to why someone is forming stones.
- *Oxalate.*   With calcium, this is the other major component of most stones.
- *Sodium.*   As discussed in Chapter 8, more sodium in your urine means an increased calcium excretion. For people who excrete too much sodium, simply lowering the amount of salt in the diet can lower urinary calcium and sometimes stop a stone problem.
- *Citrate.*   This is the best inhibitor of the calcium oxalate system. If it is low, it indicates a very good type of therapeutic intervention—*potassium citrate* supplements.
- *Phosphate.*   This may give an idea of how much protein you are eating. Also, people who excrete very large or very small amounts of phosphate may have a peculiar disorder in stone formation.
- *Uric Acid.*   This is a component of some stones. In addition, a high urinary uric acid can be part of the cause of a calcium oxalate stone.

The tests for uric acid and phosphate are costly. I like to have this information but will forgo it if economic considerations are overriding. The first five urine tests can be collected with a boric acid preservative in the collection bottle. Uric acid cannot be measured if boric acid is used.

Translating Your Workup into a Risk Assessment

The easiest way to illustrate the different risk categories is with specific examples. The following three case histories will show you people at varying risk for stone recurrence and how their risk factors determine their level of treatment and dietary regimen. (See Chapter 15 for additional case histories.)

Fever and Infection

Jean is a thirty-one-year-old woman who has passed two calcium oxalate stones. She came to my office during the second stone episode with a fever and urinary tract infection that did not respond to standard antibiotic therapy. An X ray showed a struvite stone, and urinalysis showed that she had the bacteria *Proteus* growing in her urine. After several conversations, Jean mentioned that she had lost and regained 30 pounds in the past year and that weight "cycling" was not unusual for her.

Comment: Jean had made another calcium oxalate stone that became infected with struvite. The infection caused the staghorn. The presence of a kidney infection with obstructing stones has the potential to lead to sepsis or a bloodstream infection. I was looking at a potentially life-threatening situation.

Once she is surgically rid of the current stone problem, we have to be very careful that she does not make any more stones. This last stone was particularly serious. She now requires regular comprehensive evaluations and ongoing surveillance with regular follow-up X rays.

Jean's dietary history of weight cycling reflects a stuff-fast pattern that probably caused her stone disease. She is a "high risk" individual who must follow fluid and dietary guidelines extremely carefully and cure her eating disorder. Another stone episode could be life threatening.

Lithotripsy in the Family

David is a thirty-two-year-old man who has passed six calcium oxalate stones—four during the last year and a half. The last stone became stuck in his right ureter and had to be treated with laser lithotripsy. In addition, his latest KUB film showed three more retained stones, each about 3 millimeters.

David's father and brother have both passed multiple stones.

Comment: I now have a real clinical problem. David has had a lot of trouble with his stones and still has three retained stones. Stones of 3 millimeters usually pass if they begin to move.

I am going to do a complete evaluation of this patient. His urinary chemistries will indicate if medication is needed in addition to a diet. I will certainly get follow-up KUB films, even if he is asymptomatic. If the follow-up films show stone growth while David was on a diet only, I would probably add medication. If the stones grew big enough so that I was afraid they might not pass if they started to move, I might recommend an elective ESWL treatment.

On Vacation

Robert, a twenty-three-year-old man, passed his first kidney stone in August, within two hours of the onset of colic. It was a single, 1.5-millimeter calcium oxalate stone. He had just come back from a three-week vacation at the beach. He had "gorged" on ice cream during this period and his only regularly consumed beverage was iced tea.

He has no family history of stone disease and his weight is appropriate for his build. His IVP, done after the stone passed, showed no retained stones and normal renal anatomy.

Comment: This is the mildest form of stone disease we see. Although Robert suffered two hours of colicky pain—an awful experience for anyone—he was at no risk. We also have a fairly good idea why he made his stone. It was most likely precipitated by dehydration at the beach, a high calcium intake of ice cream, a high oxalate intake of tea, and ultraviolet light exposure in the sun.

Robert was given the simple blood tests outlined earlier. I would like to evaluate his urinary chemistries, but practical and economic considerations suggest that some dietary counseling and advice about sun exposure and fluid intake might be sufficient unless he has further trouble.

Many people pass a single stone in their lives and never have another. Robert would be a "low probability" risk and treated accordingly.

Where Are You on the Risk Ladder?

I hope everyone reading this book is willing to make the dietary and lifestyle changes necessary to prevent a stone recurrence. Understanding your risk potential for another stone episode will tell you how closely you have to follow the advice in Part Two.

At High Risk

Anyone in this category must follow fluid, dietary, lifestyle, and medication guidelines to the letter. People at high risk generally have underlying medical conditions that predispose them to stone formation. Following the Master Plan outlined in Part Three may also prevent permanent kidney damage.

At Risk

This category is the largest and most difficult to monitor. Fluid guidelines must be followed carefully and specific dietary changes for your type of stone should become part of your regimen. People in this category sometimes go several years between episodes, during which time they begin to "cheat" on their diets. Each new kidney stone creates a greater chance of complication, additional need for surgical intervention, and potential kidney damage. If lifestyle changes are needed, these guidelines must be followed.

At Low Risk

If you think that you fall in this category, then basic fluid and dietary advice for your type of stone formation should be sufficient to prevent a recurrence.

If you are at *any* risk for future stone disease, the dietary and lifestyle advice in Part Two could change your life.

PART TWO

THE PLAN

Drink and dance and laugh and lie,
Love, the reeling midnight through,
For tomorrow we shall die!
(But, alas, we never do.)

—DOROTHY PARKER

14

NO MORE KIDNEY STONES

I don't want to eat a head of lettuce and a carrot for the rest of my life. I can find something I want to eat for the rest of my life but don't tell me this is it. This is crazy.

Most diets fail because they make impossible demands on the dieter. Once the offending component creeps back into the diet—whether it is salt, sugar, fat, or even solid food after a liquid weight-loss regimen—it is accompanied by the unwanted weight or medical condition.

The key to success is changing the way you think about certain foods and in finding acceptable substitutes. Our goal is to deflect certain habits that lead to stone formation rather than trying to restructure your eating patterns completely. In fact, the less you have to change, the more likely you are to continue this Plan into the future.

Diet Is Not a Four-Letter Word

Eating is one of the pleasures in life. Because a diet must necessarily restrict this enjoyment, it is important that the diet not limit you more than necessary. In many cases, eliminating the dietary and lifestyle behaviors that have triggered your stone episodes can solve the problem. While some stone sufferers will have to make more comprehensive changes to their diets, most people must focus on specific troublemakers.

We are going to recommend guidelines that will be totally compatible with any other diet you might require. In fact, many of the recommendations will reinforce aspects of other diets, such as The

American Heart Association Diet. *Any diet we give you has to make
sense for all of you, not just your kidneys.*

Some patients ask, "how much of this do I *really* have to follow?" The answer is, the more you deviate from the Plan, the more
likely you are to make a stone.

What follows is our dietary prescription. It will change your urine
volume and chemistries and minimize the chance that you will make
more stones.

The Master Plan

1. *Identify and limit particular troublemakers in the diet.* (See
Chapter 8.) These troublemakers include

> Oxalate
> Salt
> Excess calcium
> Dietary supplements (vitamins, minerals)
> Fad diets

There are a number of people who must avoid high-oxalate foods.
(See Chapter 17, "Operation Oxalate.") Particularly rich sources of
oxalate are spinach, rhubarb, tea, cocoa, nuts, nut oils, chocolate, and
berries (see the Appendix, Table 2). When you do eat foods in this
group, keep the portions small and drink extra water to "dilute the
mistake."

Avoid excess salt, as a high sodium intake can increase urinary
calcium. (See "Salt" in Chapter 8, and the Appendix, Table 4.) Salt
is a hidden ingredient in a number of foods, such as

> Soy and teriyaki sauce, catsup, mustard
> Salted snack foods (pretzels, crackers, chips)
> Canned or dehydrated soups and broths
> Sausage, bacon, frankfurters, and lunch meats
> Tomato juice, V-8 juice, and Clamato juice
> Pickles, olives, sauerkraut

As a general rule, people with calcium stones should be eating
about 800 milligrams of calcium a day. You should not be taking
unlimited amounts of dairy products or calcium supplements. Certain foods are also calcium-rich (see the Appendix, Table 3).

However, a low-calcium diet is not generally recommended, as this increases oxalate absorption and the risk for bone problems or osteoporosis. (See "The Calcium Controversy" in Chapter 8.) Discuss your particular situation with your doctor to determine the amount of calcium you should be ingesting. If you fall into a higher daily need category (e.g., teenagers, pregnant women, or elderly women), you need to consult a doctor or dietitian for specific advice.

We would prefer that you not supplement vitamin C unless your diet is particularly poor in this nutrient. Oxalate is a by-product of vitamin C metabolism (see Chapters 8 and 17), and it is therefore not recommended for stone formers.

2. *Decrease the amount of animal protein you eat and find acceptable substitutes.* Most of us eat far more protein than we need. And, as cholesterol-conscious dieters substitute chicken and fish for red meat, they are eating huge portions of white meat. Please note: Both chicken and fish are animal protein. For the purposes of kidney stone formation, the same limitations apply. (See Chapter 8.)

Ideally, you should not eat more than 3 ounces of animal protein at any one time. This is approximately the size of a single deck of cards or the palm of your hand. You should try to reduce what you eat in the evening in particular and eat more at lunchtime, keeping your daily total under 8 ounces.

It is not unusual to find a stone former who is consuming six to ten times what is needed by the body. Occasional protein intakes in excess of 8 to 10 ounces per day are tolerable. If you find yourself eating 10 to 12-ounce steaks for dinner on a regular basis, you are preparing your kidneys for a stone. (See the Appendix, Tables 5 and 6.)

When you do violate this rule, drink more fluids, and do not overindulge often.

3. *Avoid dehydration and increase fluid consumption.* A common refrain heard from stone sufferers is the difficulty in drinking enough fluids. Fluids are crucial to the Plan. You must retrain yourself to think about how much is coming *out* as opposed to how much is going *in*. (See Chapter 7 for guidelines.)

You should maintain a urine output of at least 2000 cc/day. For big men, the goal is 2500 cc (1000 cc is 1.1 quarts). If you have formed many stones, you should probably try to make 3000 cc of urine daily.

A twenty-four-hour urine output of less than a quart is not good.

If your output is 500 cc, or a pint, you have a real problem. As a rough guide, 2000 cc of urine a day means that you should urinate at least seven times a day with your bladder relatively full. And remember, every day counts. You cannot expect to boost your urinary output on weekends and avoid kidney stones.

It is impossible to tell how much fluid you will have to consume to achieve this goal. At high altitudes, when you are exercising or when it is hot, the amount of fluids you must drink will be considerably more than during a normal office routine.

Water is the best fluid to consume. (See Chapter 7 on hard and mineral water.) Certain fruit and vegetable juices are high in sodium or oxalates or can cause an acid urine. (See Chapter 5, "How and Why Kidney Stones Form.") They include

Tomato and V-8 juice (sodium)
Cranberry juice (acidic and high-oxalate)

4. *Attain and maintain a healthy weight.*   Stone disease is most often the result of eating "too well." The more overweight you are, the more waste products you produce for the kidney to excrete. Achieve and then maintain your appropriate weight. Do not eat in binges.

This is not a weight-loss plan, but the change in animal protein, fat consumption, and portion size may help you to attain a more ideal weight.

Tips for Staying on the Plan

I can kid my wife, I can kid the doctor, but I can't kid my kidney stones.

Since you cannot always follow a diet to the letter, you have to know how and when to "indulge." The amount of indulgence that will produce a stone recurrence will vary from person to person.

But do not misread this information: If you are indulging yourself once a day, every day, you are not changing your diet, you are fooling yourself. You will see the extra pounds and forbidden foods creep back—along with that awful renal colic pain.

One of my patients had a tremendous sweet tooth. In fact, he lived each day and each meal to have his dessert. At our first meeting, after he had suffered five different stone episodes, we discussed the oxalate content of his chocolate desserts. He agreed that it was important to limit his intake of chocolate—which was considerable. A year, and two more stones later, he returned and confessed.

The doctor can help you only if you admit to certain habits. This is less a confession than an honest look at the elements that are causing you to make stones. In the case of my chocoholic patient, we agreed to limiting portion sizes and to have him follow *every* chocolate dessert with two glasses of water. He has made no more stones in the past three years.

Suppose you have an Italian grandma who always serves dishes made with lots of tomato sauce. You cannot change Grandma and you can't offend her by not eating her food—if you know what's good for you. This is a situation where you refuse seconds and increase your fluid intake during and after the meal.

The extent to which you must follow these directives is based on two key questions:

1. How severe is your problem?
2. Can you be treated with dietary advice only, or do you need medication?

I find that most kidney stone sufferers are initially highly motivated; the pain of a stone episode is not easily forgotten. However, a year later, you must remember that you are a stone former when you have a steak dinner and are thinking of having chocolate mousse for dessert. How many glasses of water did you drink with dinner? And how many are you going to have to drink after dinner to flush the extra oxalates in the chocolate through your kidneys?

In the next chapters we will teach you to recognize your own danger zones and show you how to change menus, drink more fluids, and handle the events and menus of everyday life.

15

FINDING THE DIET THAT IS RIGHT FOR YOU

I need to lose 20 pounds. I have a suit sitting there waiting for a 165-pound man.

I have an eating disorder: I love to eat. I'd be 400 pounds if I could, but I can't because I would die and I don't want to do that right now.

I make my tea so dark I have to put it back in the microwave to heat it back up.

When people come to my office, we tailor a diet to each particular case. The advice will vary with the type of stone, the workup results, the risk potential for another recurrence, and the personal background of the patient. (See Chapter 13.) One person will have to avoid high-oxalate foods and vitamin supplements, whereas another will have to concentrate on controlling the amount of protein in the diet.

Since we cannot do the same analysis for everyone reading this book, this chapter contains specific information to help you recognize the troublemakers in your own diet and adapt the Master Plan to your own type of stone problem.

Rating Yourself

The first thing you must do is determine which parts of the Master Plan to focus on. You should think of it as a rating scale of 0 to 4:

0 — of no consequence to your specific stone disease
1 — of minor consequence
2 — pay attention to these items
3 — important to limit/change
4 — crucial to limit/change

If you rate a 4 on any particular food or lifestyle element, you must make immediate, permanent changes to these aspects of your diet and life if you are to avoid a kidney stone recurrence. A 3 also indicates a need for change and careful limitation of the offending element. A 1 or 2 indicates a watchful eye and extra fluids to wash away any extra indulgence. Don't worry about trying to pinpoint yourself on this rating scale. It is only a guide to indicate which parts of the Master Plan you need to emphasize.

You must distinguish between your day-to-day routine and unusual situations or behavior. If you make kidney stones only at certain times of the year (e.g., on vacation when your fluid intake is limited, changed, or sweated away), then you must adjust your fluid intake and diet on these occasions.

How Much Do You Have to Change?

Not every stone former has to make radical dietary changes. It is possible that your kidney stones may have been triggered by a single food and/or event. Some simple detective work may uncover a single glaringly obvious "offender" that could be easily eliminated from the diet—and thereby resolve the problem.

In other cases, you will need only to increase your fluid consumption under circumstances where you have been "running dry."

However, most stone disease is not eliminated quite that easily.

Do You Consume Too Many Troublemakers?

The following questions will help you analyze the key troublemakers in your diet. These questions are not designed as an exact measure of the foods in your diet but only to start you thinking about the amount of these substances that you are consuming.

Oxalates

This rating is important for people with calcium oxalate stones.

1. Do you drink hot tea after every meal or quarts of iced tea in the summer?
2. Do you steep your tea until it is black?
3. Do you prefer hot chocolate or cocoa over coffee?
4. Do you eat Italian food at least three times a week or dishes with lots of tomato sauce?
5. Do you eat Chinese food cooked in peanut oil often?
6. Do you snack on peanut butter and jelly sandwiches?
7. Do you include spinach in your weekly diet because you were told green leafy vegetables are very healthy?
8. Do you look forward to summer because it is strawberry and raspberry season?
9. Do you sprinkle wheat bran on your cereal to boost the fiber content of your diet?
10. Do you consume large servings of legumes and soy products in your diet?

Rating: Using the oxalate tables in the Appendix, you can accurately measure the amount of high-oxalate foods you consume daily. Vegetarians, health food advocates, heavy tea or cocoa drinkers, summer fruit bingers, and heavy tomato sauce eaters probably rate a 3 to 4 in this category. (See Chapter 17, "Operation Oxalate.")

Sodium

This rating is important for people with calcium oxalate stones. Sodium is an especially critical part of the Master Plan if your doctor has told you that your urinary calcium excretion is high. (See Chapter 8 on the relation of sodium and calcium.)

1. Do you always add salt to your food, even before tasting it?
2. Do you frequently eat cold breakfast cereals other than puffed rice, puffed wheat, and shredded wheat?
3. Do you snack on potato chips, corn or tortilla chips, crackers, pretzels, and popcorn?

4. Do you usually consume the following for lunch?
   Lunch meats like bologna, salami, and ham
   Hot dogs
   Canned soups
5. Do you add the following in cooking or at the table?
   Salt
   Flavoring salts (garlic and onion)
   Soy sauce

Rating: If you *always* salt your food, regularly eat the first two
items in question (3) or a great deal of Asian foods (soy), and lunch
at least twice a week on cured meats or canned soup, you probably
rate a 4. You are probably a 2 to 3 if you prefer savory tastes to sweet
ones and eat a fair amount of salty foods. Many people consume
large amounts of hidden salt in prepared foods. This is not a prescription for a low-salt diet: You can go too far if you eliminate all salt.

Vitamin and Mineral Supplements

This rating is important for people with calcium oxalate stones.

1. Do you take the following?
   Multivitamins with minerals
   Vitamin C
   Vitamin D
   Fish-liver oil
   Mineral supplements containing calcium
2. Do you look through the displays of vitamins and minerals at a
   health food store or drugstore and try different products?
3. Do you feel that your diet needs a vitamin or mineral supplement, and do you try products suggested by helpful friends and
   relatives?

Rating: This is a fairly straightforward rating. If you take more
than 1500 milligrams of vitamin C daily, you certainly get a 4. Smaller
amounts may give you a 2 or 3.
   Vitamin D supplements (found in fish-liver oils) can be important in causing stones. The more you take, the higher your rating
here. Calcium supplements depend on your total calcium intake. (See
"Calcium," following, and in Chapter 8.)

Calcium

Contrary to popular belief, excess calcium is only occasionally the culprit in stone disease. (See Chapter 8 on Hypercalciuria.) This rating is important for people with calcium stones *who have been tested as overabsorbers of calcium.*

1. Do you usually drink or use in cooking more than three servings of milk a day?
2. Do you frequently eat the following desserts: ice cream, ice milk, frozen yogurt, frozen dessert Tofutti (soy-based)?
3. Do you use the following cheese for snacks or sandwiches?
   American, Brie, Cheddar, cream cheese, feta, Monterey Jack, Swiss
   Low-sodium, low-fat cheeses, Dorman's light, Weight Watchers brand
4. Do you use the following in cooking or in mixed dishes you prepare or order out?
   American, Brie, Cheddar, cream cheese, feta, Monterey Jack, Swiss, mozzarella
   Part-skim or skim-milk mozzarella, light cream cheese, Weight Watchers cheeses
5. Do you eat the following at least once a week?
   Sardines
   Canned Salmon
   Oysters
   Tofu
6. Do you consume the following foods that are fortified with calcium?
   Orange juice
   Cold breakfast cereals
   Instant oatmeal
   Tums/Rolaids

Rating: If you are taking large amounts of calcium-containing antacids, plus a moderately high dairy intake, you may get a 4. If you eat large amounts of calcium in two to three of the categories listed you probably rate a 2 or 3. Some people mistakenly believe that low-fat dairy products are also low in calcium. This is incorrect. You should not, however, try to eliminate calcium-containing foods without consulting a doctor. (See "The Calcium Controversy" in Chapter 8.)

Weight Loss or Gain

This rating is important for anyone who periodically gains and/or loses 10 or more pounds or uses fad diets to lose weight.

1. Have you had a weight loss or gain in the past six months of more than 5 pounds?
2. Have you used liquid protein regimens to lose weight?
3. Have you gone on a high-protein diet to lose weight?
4. Do you exercise vigorously (and perspire a lot) along with weight-reduction programs?

Rating: Rapid weight loss can cause kidney stones (see Chapter 10). Anyone with a weight swing of 10 pounds or more within a three- to six-month period probably rates a 4. This rating goes down with the amount of weight lost per week. If you are losing more than 1 to 2 pounds a week for a sustained period of time, you must slow this loss if you are to control your stone-forming potential. Any large weight swing should be considered a potential troublemaker.

How to Know If You Are Eating
Too Much Protein

Rating the amount of protein in your diet is important for uric acid and calcium stone formers. Chances are, if you have made stones, you are consuming more protein than you require.

Protein Consumption Survey

1. Do you order three-egg omelets with ham, bacon, or cheese for breakfast?
2. Do you enjoy deli sandwiches that you can hardly fit your mouth around?
3. When you go out for dinner, do you have second helpings of meat, fish, or poultry?
4. Do you go to "all-you-can-eat" buffets and load up on cold cuts, meats, and fish?

5. Do you go out for fast food frequently and order the biggest burger on the menu?
6. Do you go to seafood restaurants that serve unlimited amounts of shrimp, crab, or lobster?
7. Do you have a late-night snack of a thick meat sandwich?
8. In a typical day, including all meals and snacks, how many ounces of meat, cheese, fish, and poultry do you consume?
    11 or more ounces a day
    7 to 10 ounces a day
    4 to 6 ounces a day

Rating: If you normally eat 12 ounces of steak at a meal, consider yourself a "meat-and-potatoes" person, go back for seconds and thirds at a buffet or "all-you-can-eat" restaurant, or eat large sandwiches, you are probably a protein glutton. You are in trouble at a 4.

If you eat sensibly during the week and then eat four pieces of chicken at a weekend barbecue or party or three 8-ounce hamburgers, you need to rein in your protein consumption. You are probably a 2 or 3 during the week and a 4 on the weekend.

How Much Is Too Much?

Most people eat more animal protein than they need. The RDA (Recommended Daily Allowance) of protein for healthy adults is 0.8 grams of protein per kilogram of body weight. (See the Appendix for conversion tables and protein/body weight tables.) For example, a 70-kilogram (154-pound) man should ideally consume 56 grams of protein a day (0.8 x 70 kg = 56 g protein per day) to satisfy his protein requirements. This translates into roughly 7 to 8 ounces of meat daily.

A young athlete in training may need up to 1.5 grams of protein per kilogram per day. This translates into 105 grams or three 8-ounce servings of meat daily for a 70-kilogram male. This is almost double the amount of the RDA for healthy adults. But the most active young athletes are a very special case.

If we were setting up a perfect diet for a stone former, it would include no more than 3 ounces of protein at each meal. If you are in the "high risk" category, you should follow this recommendation. We are not as concerned with those stone formers eating 10 to 20 percent more protein than they need as we are with those eating 100 percent more than the RDA of protein.

Portion Sizes

Let's put all this in terms that may be easier to understand. One 3-ounce serving of meat looks like

The palm of a hand
A deck of cards
A cassette
A mayonnaise lid

In terms of "real food" this amount is equal to

1 medium pork chop
$^1/_2$ of a whole chicken breast
1 unbreaded fish fillet
1 fast-food hamburger

Most people can relate to a generic fast-food hamburger. This hamburger weighs about 3 ounces and contains 12.5 grams of protein. If all of your protein for a day is three "hamburger equivalents," you are within a reasonable protein range. If you are up to five or six, you are well over the acceptable amount. We actually find that some stone formers are consuming as much meat as would be found in twenty "fast-food hamburger equivalents."

Finally, if you eat carefully during the week and binge on the weekends, you may still be in trouble. Remember, one half-pound hamburger (the home barbecue size) may be equal to all of your daily protein needs.

When you overdo protein at one party buffet, you can "dilute the mistake" by drinking a lot of water. When you are two to three times over your ideal protein consumption for your weight on a regular basis, you must change your habits.

How to Know If You Are Drinking Enough Fluids

This rating is important for every stone type. There is no simpler form of therapy for stone disease.

Fluid Consumption Survey

1. How much do you consume?
       1 to 6 glasses (8 oz) of fluids
       6 to 12 glasses
       12 to 16 glasses
2. When do you cut back on fluids?
       At work
       During certain activities (e.g., skiing)
       On dates
       When there is no bathroom readily available
       Not consciously, at all
3. What is your alcoholic beverage consumption?
       1 or more drinks a day
       3 to 6 drinks a week
       1 or 2 drinks a week
       None, or less than 1 a week

Rating: If your habitual urinary volume is in the neighborhood of 500 cc, or only half a quart, fluids get a 4 in importance. If your stone episodes have correlated with situations when you have been prone to dehydration, such as a vacation in Arizona, fluids also get a 4 for these special times.

If you have an unusual stone-forming process such as cystinuria, increasing your urinary output is the most important change you have to make.

As we have pointed out many times, it is not what goes in that is important but what comes out. Therefore, the question should be: How do I know if I am drinking enough fluid to produce at least 2000 cc a day of urine? If you have collected a twenty-four-hour urine, you have some idea what this volume means. If you have not, on a day when you are home, you might try seeing how long it takes you to fill a quart container. Remember that our goal is somewhat above 2 quarts.

The official recommendation of the National Kidney Foundation is 2500 cc a day. Many people will not reach this goal. It is certainly optimal. If you are at 400 cc and go to 1500 cc, that improvement will have a greater effect than if you are at 1500 cc and go to 2500 cc.

More important, are there days when you fall below 200 cc because of special circumstances? Drinking the fluid equivalent of seven 8-ounce glasses of water, in addition to the fluid that is normally in food, will just barely get you to our goal on a quiet day at home when the weather is not too hot and the air in your house is not too dry. The same seven glasses will not put you close to our goal in the middle of a cold Vermont winter when the heat is on all of the time and the air is dry, or if you are perspiring on a hot July day. Moreover, if you have a diarrheal problem, you must offset the fluid losses in your stool. (See Chapter 7.)

You must become conscious of the approximate amount of urine you form, and you must have a general understanding of how often you need to urinate to reach the urinary output goal of 2000 cc.

Some of you will reach the 2000 cc goal on most days. *Do not become complacent.*

Do You Weigh Too Much?

This category is one that you should discuss with your own doctor. Desirable weights vary by bone size and muscle-to-fat ratios. Stone formers need to look at their weight in relation to the foods they eat that have caused them to gain weight (e.g., excess protein) and the types of diets they go on to lose it (e.g., quick weight loss).

Rating: Binge eaters and fad dieters rate a 4 in this category. People who are 20 or more pounds overweight probably rate a 2 to 3 if they go on and off various diets.

Food Diary

If you are still not sure of the source of your dietary problem, or if you would like a fuller analysis of your own eating patterns, a food diary may show you where you are adding the ingredients that contribute to kidney stones. It is a revealing exercise if done properly.

In the Appendix there is a blank food diary along with two sample food diaries showing a good day's food intake and a bad day's. These sample diaries include breakfast, midmorning snack, lunch, midafternoon snack, dinner, and late-night snacks.

You can submit your food diary to a registered dietitian for a nutritional analysis. Or you can tally the information by using the charts provided in the Appendix to calculate the important nutrients that influence stone formation.

Classic Stone-Forming Profiles

While a food diary may uncover your own eating patterns, you can also use the following case histories to help identify some classic stone-forming profiles that may fit your own.

The Young Male Milk Drinker

Robert is a trim, twenty-three-year-old man who is often described as "wholesome as apple pie."

Breakfast is commonly bacon and eggs, toast and butter, and a large glass of whole milk. Lunches are frequently eaten on the run in fast-food places and consist of a cheeseburger and fries topped off with a large milkshake. An afternoon snack of donuts and milk is not unusual.

Robert dislikes coffee and does not drink hard liquor. He plays on the company baseball team once a week and, on these occasions, may indulge in a few beers with the team.

He is a "meat-and-potatoes-man" for dinner, with milk as the beverage of choice. The last thing at night might be cookies and more milk.

Between the cheeses in his entrées, the ice cream on weekends, and the whole milk as his beverage, he has tipped the calcium balance in favor of forming three calcium oxalate stones.

The Plan: Robert is, most likely, the classic hyperabsorber of calcium who needs to decrease his calcium intake. He must learn to replace the large quantities of dairy products he consumes with other fluids such as fruit juices and water. He must have a *maximum* of three servings of dairy products a day. He must not fall into the trap of reducing his calcium too drastically, though, as this may increase his oxalate excretion. (See Chapter 8.)

He must also try to balance his diet with more fruits and vegetables while being careful not to include the oxalate-rich ones.

After physical activities, he must drink extra water or other liquids and avoid too much of dehydrating alcoholic beverages like beer.

Master Plan

1. Troublemakers
         Calcium   4
         Salt   2
2. Protein Consumption   2
3. Fluid Consumption   2
4. Weight   –

The Protein Glutton

*I'm my own worst enemy. I'll be good for six months, run
in marathons, lose weight. Then I'll go back and put on
40 or 50 pounds.*

Chet is an overweight, forty-eight-year-old businessman in a high-stress
position. He is 5 feet 8 inches tall and weighs 180 pounds. His "spare
tire" seems to spread a little more each year. Between the pressures of
his job and his family responsibilities, he finds little time in his schedule to eat three square meals a day or to exercise.

He has little time for or interest in breakfast, which is usually a cup
of coffee. When he gets to the office, he often has a donut and a second
cup of coffee.

There is no time to leave his desk for lunch, so he usually orders
in a lean corned beef or roast beef sandwich that weighs in at half a
pound. He enjoys the sour pickle on the side and often asks for an extra.
His favorite drink is a large bottle of Snapple Iced Tea. The afternoon
is spent tied to the desk where he may have another Snapple.

After his last promotion, he started eating dinner out three or four
times a week at a "good" restaurant. To unwind, he orders a cocktail
at the bar and tosses down a few handfuls of mixed salted nuts. With
a full three- to four-course dinner, he drinks wine. After a stressful day,
no thought is given to deprivation or dieting; a bountiful dinner is his
personal reward. He normally eats a large prime cut of meat. It may be
beef, lamb, or pork—it does not matter as long as it is a large portion.
He enjoys well-prepared vegetables. After dinner comes dessert and a
cup of tea, since coffee keeps him up at night.

One year after being promoted, Chet gained an additional 10 pounds
and developed a mixed stone composed of calcium oxalate and uric
acid.

The Plan: Chet is a protein glutton. He likes his meat and he likes large amounts of it. He must reduce his total protein consumption by controlling the portion size of his meat servings and trying alternative menu choices in this food group. His weight should naturally fall when his portions are reduced.

The sodium content of his diet is also unusually high due to the cured meats, pickles, nuts, and other convenience foods he often consumes. Avoiding these foods will have the double benefit of lowering both the sodium and oxalate content of his diet.

He must remember to include two servings of low-fat dairy products, which he could accomplish by having skim milk with cereal for breakfast or a low-fat yogurt. Replacing his morning donut with a healthy breakfast is also desirable. Most important, he must increase his fluid consumption with water or other healthy fluids in place of the tea he is drinking.

Master Plan

1. Troublemakers
   - Oxalate   1
   - Salt   3
2. Protein   4
3. Fluid   2
4. Weight   3

The Uric Acid Stone Former

Peter is a sixty-year-old Eastern European man who has non-insulin-dependent diabetes and gout. He is 5 foot 7 inches tall and weighs 170 pounds. His diet reflects both his ethnic background and the all-American good life. It is laden with fat and salty foods.

Breakfast is coffee with milk, fried eggs and salami, and bagel with cream cheese. A weekend luncheon spread may be a variety of appetizers like herring in cream sauce, sardines, and smoked fish. A redeeming salad of fresh lettuce, tomato, cucumber, and sliced onion is a part of the meal plan. He likes to swim on the weekends.

Dinner is heavy with homemade chicken soup as a first course, chopped liver as an appetizer, and a main course of potted meat (pot roasts, brisket, flanken) in a rich gravy in which potatoes and vegetables have been added. Dessert is often sponge cake and two cups of tea. He eats many stews, potted meats, and heavily sauced fish and vegetables.

The Plan: Peter's diet is loaded with high-purine foods. (See the Appendix and Chapter 8 on purines and uric acid.) Although he can still eat familiar meat, fish, and poultry items, they must be prepared in a way that eliminates the purine-laden gravies and sauces. His food should be baked, broiled, or microwaved. He must also lower the fat content of his food to achieve and maintain a lower weight for his height. This will improve both of his medical conditions.

Master Plan

1. Troublemakers
        Salt   3
        Oxalate   2
        Special Note: Gravy   4
2. Protein   3
3. Fluid   2
4. Weight   2

"Susan"

Susan is a twenty-four-year-old female who had passed two stones. She is 5 feet 4 inches tall and weighs 115 pounds. When she came to me she had no particular dietary habits that seemed out of the ordinary. In other words, she was already an atypical stone former. When her stones were analyzed, they contained half calcium oxalate and half apatite. Her blood bicarbonate level was 20 (normal is above 24).

The Plan: I immediately suspected that she might have a disorder of renal acid-base regulation. Testing proved that she did have renal tubular acidosis of a mild form. She has been taking potassium citrate now for four years and has not made another stone.

Master Plan

1. Troublemakers
        Susan's problem is not her diet, but she must keep her fluid volume up.

Crohn's Case History

When you bring up a child, they always say "eat plenty of greens." Now they say don't eat certain greens. What's right and what's wrong?

George had a bowel resection for Crohn's disease ten years ago and had 8 feet of intestine removed. At 5 feet 10 inches tall and 210 pounds, he is overweight. His cholesterol is low (partially due to the rapid transit of fat through his remaining intestine), and he feels no compunction to watch his fat or egg intake. He has six to eight bowel movements a day.

George runs a consulting business and travels extensively. He is often very hungry in the morning and has buttered rolls, sausages rolled in bread, and strong tea. Because of his long hours, he had a kitchen built into his office and there are always chocolates, cookies, and chips lying around. He will often eat an entire box of chocolate biscuits or the entire bag of chips if he has skipped lunch. When he does eat lunch, it usually consists of pizza or a snack of whatever is left over in the kitchen.

George eats out a lot. His wife has urged him to switch to fish and chicken as she feels they are healthier for him, but he prefers steak. She has also tried to have him switch to low-fat chips and cookies, but he feels that they taste like cardboard and are not worth eating.

When first diagnosed with kidney stone disease, he was given a list of high-oxalate foods and told to avoid them. He finds the advice contradictory to the current emphasis on greens and fresh fruit and vegetables.

The Plan: George must control three things: his weight; his fat intake, which is driving the diarrhea; and his oxalate intake. Anyone with this number of bowel movements does not have bowel disease under control: The diarrhea is too frequent.

The first step in trying to reduce his bowel movements each day is to put more soluble fiber in his diet such as bananas, apples, and oatmeal. This fiber is a useful means of controlling diarrhea. He may need small amounts of immodium. He must increase fluids to replace what is being lost in diarrhea and avoid alcohol and nuts.

By decreasing the fat in his diet, he will also have an easier time controlling his weight.

Finally, anyone with bowel disease must watch oxalates carefully. (See Chapter 9 and the Appendix for oxalate-rich foods.)

Master Plan

1. Troublemakers
       Oxalate   4
       Salt   2
       Alcohol   1
2. Protein   2
3. Fluid   3
4. Weight   2

Yo-Yo Dieting or Weight Cycling

Ralph is a sixty-year-old man who has passed at least a dozen stones. Two of them were analyzed; one contained pure uric acid and the other was a mixed calcium–uric acid stone. He has a chronic problem with his weight. At 5 feet 11 inches, he ideally should weigh about 185 pounds. During the past ten years his weight has varied between 195 and 230. Most of his episodes of renal colic have followed periods of rapid weight loss. In the past, he has used liquid protein diets to effect weight loss.

His wife makes sure that he drinks fluids whenever possible, but he feels that too much water bloats his body.

The Plan: Ralph's is a common and difficult problem. He should learn to eat less and to maintain a relatively constant weight in the 180s. However, he is probably going to have a chronic weight problem. That is not to say that various behavioral approaches should not be tried to help him. However, until the scientists learn how to control this type of weight problem, the nephrologists are stuck with trying to prevent such people from making stones. What do we do? First, we encourage the person to use a scale to monitor weight loss and not to lose more than 1 to 2 pounds per week. We emphasize the need to maintain a urinary output of no less than 2000 cc a day, and we encourage more.

Finally, doctors frequently give alkaline potassium salts such as K-lyte (not K-lyte Cl), Polycitra K, and Urocit K. These all require prescriptions and should be given under a doctor's direction. Sometimes, as outlined in Chapter 10 ("Dieting Your Way to a Kidney Stone"), doctors will also give sodium bicarbonate. (See Chapter 24, "Medications.")

You can lose weight safely if you have made stones, but you are at risk of forming more stones if you do not take proper precautions and set safe and realistic weight-loss goals.

Master Plan

1. Troublemakers
        Liquid Protein Diet   4
2. Protein   3
3. Fluids   3
4. Weight   3

The Problems of a "Healthy Diet"

Sonia, a fifty-something woman, is extremely well read regarding the contents of the foods she eats. Although she feels that she needs to lose the weight she has put on since menopause, she has cultivated what the current press would call a "healthy diet." It includes low-fat cereal in the morning with skim milk and fruit and a cranberry drink at the office. Lunch is often a Greek salad, where she restricts some of the feta cheese, or a health-salad sandwich on seven-grain bread with mayonnaise or mustard, cheese, sprouts, avocados, and shredded carrots. She will order a chocolate chip biscotti to go with this lunch because she works at a high-stress firm and feels she needs a little treat midday.

She rarely eats meat of any kind unless she is out for dinner, and she has pasta marinara that she makes for her husband several times a week. If Sonia eats a big lunch, she will eat a very light dinner and is often hungry by 9 P.M. At this point she heads for something chocolate. One favorite is raspberry sorbet with mini-chocolate morsels sprinkled on top or a Weight Watchers fudge pop. She will often buy pints of berries and eat them all.

She is also a large vitamin taker. She starts with Centrum and adds 1000 units of calcium citrate, 1000 units of vitamin C, and 400 units of vitamin E. She is asthmatic and takes Ventolin twice a day, which makes her thirsty. She often keeps hot apple cider and mulled cranberry juice on her desk in winter or iced tea in summer.

Besides a fondness for chocolate she loves salt, lemon, and vinegary tastes.

The Plan: Sonia eats a supposedly healthful diet that is extremely oxalate- and vitamin-rich. Unfortunately, she has taken the ingestion of these substances to excess. The combination of Greek salads (grape leaves are extremely high in oxalates), chocolate at night, tomato sauce several times a week, and large doses of vitamin C has pushed her oxalate levels over the top. Her "healthful" diet is actually the opposite for a stone former.

Sonia needs to cut back on tea and cranberry juice and start drinking water. Because of her knowledge of the vitamin and mineral content of food, she should be able to eat a balanced, healthy diet and eliminate many of the supplemental vitamins.

Since her taste runs to vinegary, salty foods, she needs to balance these with water and nonoxalate choices.

Master Plan

1. Troublemakers
        Vitamin supplements   3
        Oxalate   4
2. Protein   0
3. Fluids   1
4. Weight   1

Cystinuria

I was unwilling to make changes. I guess that's why there are surgeons . . .

Terry, a forty-something woman, has had kidney stones since junior high school. Her cystinuria was finally properly diagnosed when she was in college. She had her first surgery in college and has had five more since then. She takes Thiola to reduce her cystine excretion.

She is a successful businesswoman, trim, athletic, and extremely active. Because of a hectic business schedule and distaste for restaurant bathrooms, she has always found it difficult to drink the amount of fluids the doctor insists upon. As she states: "It's fine to put it in, but you've got to find a place to get rid of it."

She was extremely surprised to hear that the iced tea she was drinking was high in oxalates and not an acceptable fluid replacement for water.

The Plan: The treatment for people with cystinuria is quite focused. They must drink copious amounts of water and nonoxalate fluids to continually flush out the kidneys. While this is often described to me as a "life sentence," it is the only way to combat the stone disease in these people. They must use every trick and opportunity to get eighteen to twenty glasses of water into their system every day.

Master Plan

1.	Troublemakers	
	Tea	2
2.	Protein	0
3.	Fluid	4
4.	Weight	0

The Workaholic with Acid Indigestion

I don't like the taste of hamburgers, I like the taste of catsup. My biggest thing as a kid was mustard and catsup sandwiches.

Gerry, a forty-year-old man, often says that "sleep is not one of the things on my schedule." Traveling back and forth to Europe every third week, he grabs many meals on the run or, conversely, at good restaurants.

He has suffered from gas and heartburn since he was in high school. Although he does not have ulcers, almost everything he eats upsets his stomach. He has taken Zantac, Tums, Rolaids, and different natural products to try to eliminate a pain that often feels like "a heart attack."

Gerry is a lazy eater: If something is in the refrigerator or on his plate, he'll eat it. On his own he prefers sliced steak, hamburger, or chicken doused in catsup or dressing. He actually prefers the taste of catsup to the hamburger he puts it on. He eats a lot of fried food and feels that low-fat cheese and "guiltless" chips are not worth eating.

He feels that a meal isn't over unless he's had dessert—that includes the apple turnover at McDonald's or chocolate mousse with raspberries at a fine French restaurant.

When he's in a restaurant, he'll drink "all the water they'll give me," but he usually drinks cola when traveling or in the office. His normal day consists of no breakfast, a fast-food lunch or sandwich, and a heavy dinner. He'll snack between dinner and bedtime when at home and prefers salty treats. He is an admitted salt fanatic. His cholesterol is very high. It has dropped when he has taken up an exercise regime in conjunction with a diet several times over the past ten years.

Because of his exhausting schedule, Gerry has frequent colds. Right before his last attack, his girlfriend talked him into large doses of vitamin C to keep him healthy.

The Plan: Gerry has a combination "troublemaker" problem that consists of excessive calcium from the antacids he consumes as well as excess fat, vitamin C, and salt, which raises his oxalate excretion. His love of catsup puts additional salt and oxalate through his system regularly. In addition, he has weight swings that put excess waste into his system periodically.

Master Plan

1. Troublemakers
      Oxalates   (tomatoes—crratic)
      Calcium   3
      Vitamin C   3
      Salt   3
2. Protein   2
3. Fluids   erratic
4. Weight   2

16

LIFESTYLES OF THE KIDNEY STONE FORMER

My diet changed on that trip to Italy, I do admit to that, but I've always gotten away with it. Well, almost always.

We ski in the winter—it's cold and going to the bathroom literally means getting undressed, what with the one-piece jumpsuit . . . so I wait . . . all day if necessary.

There are certain occupations and lifestyles that may aid and abet a tendency toward kidney stones. Recognizing and adjusting to these lifestyle factors is every bit as important as modifying your diet.

The lifestyle factors contributing to stone disease include

- Bathroom access
- Situations that make you lose fluids
- Ultraviolet (UV) light exposure
- Eating patterns
- Changes in lifestyle

Bathroom Access

I have seen people make kidney stones simply because they had a low urine flow due to their difficulty in finding a convenient place to urinate. I have seen a schoolteacher who "could not excuse himself from the room during a lecture," a trader of gold futures who was afraid to leave the "pits" for fear of missing a crucial change in the market, a heart surgeon who would not leave the operating room during long critical procedures, and a secretary who had a broken bathroom at work that forced everyone to go to another floor. In the last case, the woman's lack of bathroom access led to more than a workers' compensation problem. I treated one high-steel worker who formed stones because he consciously restricted his liquids to avoid urinating all day. His twenty-four-hour urinary volume was only 250 cc. He told me: "I love it up there—I hate to come down. I stay up all day, and you know you can't pee in the breeze."

While this last case is extreme, there are many people who consciously or unconsciously restrict fluids with the same result.

The Weary Traveler

I've been in just about every airport in the United States.

Frank, a fifty-year-old man, sold toys. He boasted that he had been in every airport in the United States with more than ten scheduled flights a day. He spent more than half of his working days traveling. He passed the first of his eight stones about three months after he began his present job. He came to my office after a stone became caught in a ureter and had to be removed via a cystoscopic procedure. The stone was calcium oxalate.

Frank admitted that he would frequently go all day without any fluids. He acquired this habit of "running dry" to avoid the need for access to a bathroom. He thought that he often urinated less than a pint a day.

Comment: Frank's twenty-four-hour urine collection while he was at home revealed nothing to explain his stone formation, but a history of his habits pointed at "bathroom access" as the culprit. We worked out a plan for him to increase his fluids that included consciously drinking several glasses of water whenever he knew he was "safe": for example, when he had checked into his final destination for the day. He also learned that getting up from his seat on an airplane to use the bathroom was not as inconvenient as his frequent trips to the emergency room.

Sharon

Sharon, a thirtyish woman, suffered from recurrent urinary tract infections, constipation, and kidney stones. She grew up in a family with three brothers and had to share one toilet with them. Her early access to the bathroom was limited. Even after she went away to school, her aversion to using the bathroom persisted. She came to me after a particularly bad urinary infection had complicated a stone episode. After we finally subdued the infection, she had to confront the possibility of kidney damage if she had a stone recurrence.

Comment: Some of you may laugh when you read about Sharon. But, if my experience is representative, at least 10 percent of the people reading this book will recognize that bathroom access has played a major role in causing their stone formation. With Sharon, solving her bathroom aversion was the key to managing both her recurrent urinary tract infections and her stones. Do not be nervous about discussing this question openly with your physician.

Fluid Loss

Any activity that makes you perspire heavily is a potential kidney stone trigger. In a dry climate, you may be unaware of how much fluid you are actually losing through your skin because it evaporates so quickly. I have treated soldiers stationed in hot climates, new joggers, a pizza maker, and people who exercise heavily and/or regularly. You must not only replace lost fluids but *drink enough to continue urinating a minimum of 2000 cc per day.* It is common for people who are sweating heavily to drink an extra glass or two of water and still urinate very little. Review the cautions in Chapter 7.

Ultraviolet (UV) Light Exposure

UV, or ultraviolet, light striking your skin initiates a chemical reaction that makes vitamin D. The amount of vitamin D formed is greater in light-colored skin than in darker or tanned skin. An excessive amount of vitamin D in the skin will cause an increased absorption of calcium in the intestine in everyone. (See Chapter 8.) In stone formers, this increase is frequently much more than in non–stone formers. Therefore, sun exposure can aggravate a stone-forming tendency. This is particularly true if the UV light exposure is acute, as in the case of winter vacationers in the tropics. Furthermore, the dehydration caused by sun exposure only aggravates the situation.

When tanning salons came into fashion, I treated a woman whose stone disease was triggered by continued UV light exposure in January.

Eating Patterns

Some people eat three square meals a day. Others eat lightly during the day and have their main meal at night, close to their bedtime. This late-night eating is conducive to the formation of kidney stones.

Jimmy

I don't have time to eat before 9 P.M. . . .

Jimmy is a fortyish man who started a new business several years ago and works sixteen-hour days in order to make it successful. He is moderately overweight for his height but plans to lose the weight as soon as he has "enough time to start exercising again." Growing up he never ate dinner before 8 P.M. and this is a habit he finds hard to break, especially given his work schedule. He has passed three kidney stones in the past five years, each time after a major presentation for new business.

Client dinners are a must and normally begin with a long cocktail hour. While he does not consider himself a heavy drinker, Jimmy is, by his own definition, "in training" and can easily put away a couple of cocktails, several glasses of wine, and a brandy or two without "losing touch." He prefers red meat but has switched to fish and chicken at his wife's insistence. After his first two stones, which were mixed uric acid and calcium oxalate, he also watches the high-oxalate foods and has cut back his chocolate and tea consumption, which were high.

Comment: Jimmy is on the right track regarding oxalates, but he has not addressed the other major factors in his stone disease: alcohol-induced dehydration and eating the main meal late at night. As explained in Chapter 8, alcohol slows the kidney's ability to excrete uric acid. Jimmy would have cocktails, a big protein dinner (fish and chicken are animal protein), and wine and then go to sleep dehydrated by the alcohol. By bedtime, the kidney must excrete all the waste products from dinner, including the backlog of uric acid, in a very small volume of urine. Since part of the sleep mechanism is to slow urine flow (perhaps allowing us to sleep), this is a time when a perfect stone-forming potential exists. And that is what was happening to Jimmy. Our plan for him was to move part of his protein consumption to lunch, cut back on alcohol and be sure to chase it with a glass of water (one for each cocktail), control portion size at night, and maintain the oxalate watch. Jimmy's triggers were directly related to his lifestyle.

Change in Lifestyle

People who move to a hot or dry climate are at an increased risk of stone formation. The move may occur because of relocation or even retirement.

Barry

Barry, a fiftyish male, retired to a house by the ocean and spent most of his time playing golf, on the beach, or helping friends with home improvement projects. He formed his first stone in twenty years after several weeks of golf and beach activities in 90°F weather. He felt that he had been drinking extra liquid but admitted that he actually urinated less and didn't bother to replace fluids while doing home improvement projects or on the beach. And, beer was often the replacement fluid. He had also been "snacking" more than usual on salty foods.

Comment: Barry's changed lifestyle is directly related to his stone attack. Long days of UV light exposure, dehydration at the beach, and doing physical activities in hot weather caused him to "run dry." His dietary prescription consists mainly of fluids. We would also recommend watching and reducing the consumption of high-oxalate foods, salt, and protein. Nevertheless, once his fluid output is raised to 2000 to 2500 cc per day on a regular basis, his stone problem should be controlled.

Although you cannot always separate dietary and lifestyle factors, there are many stone formers who must look as closely at the way they live and the things they do as at their diet.

17

OPERATION OXALATE

How do I explain oxalate to my friends?

Oxalate is a throwaway product that the body excretes in the urine. (See also Chapters 4 and 8.) It has no known function in animals. However, it is an ingredient of approximately two-thirds of all kidney stones and a key troublemaker that many people have difficulty in understanding.

Why Dietary Oxalate Is Important

All stone formers must mind their oxalate intake because, even if you've never made a calcium oxalate stone, this substance can adhere to almost any other type of stone. Some of you are going to have to be particularly careful about oxalate, especially those who have

- Bowel disease and/or chronic diarrhea
- Stone formation that began with specific high-oxalate intake (e.g., the tea drinker or the vitamin C popper)
- *Hyperoxaluria* (an uncommon genetic defect, see Chapter 4)

If your stone problem is related to the overabsorption of oxalate, the information in this chapter is especially important to your diet. There are four sources for the oxalate that appears in your urine:

- The waste products of animal protein
- Excess amounts of vitamin C
- The waste products of general metabolism
- Plant foods

131

Oxalate itself is found only in plant foods, and the highest concentrations are in dark green, leafy vegetables such as spinach, and in rhubarb, chocolate, tea, okra, nuts, beans, beets, wheat bran, and strawberries. (See the appendix, Table 2.)

The Problem with Oxalate Recommendations

There are three problems with dietary oxalate recommendations.

1. *Oxalate is difficult to measure in both food and body fluids.* Therefore, accurate and complete data are simply not available. For example, grapefruit juice has appeared on high-oxalate lists in the past. However, newer methods of measuring oxalate indicate that the older data were wrong. In fact, more recent studies have suggested that citrus fruits may reduce stone risk slightly by raising urinary citrate (a natural inhibitor). Citrus juices are therefore no longer on "to avoid" lists. However, citrus *peel* is high in oxalate.

2. *The oxalate content of food can vary greatly from one batch of a given food to another.* It is believed that aging increases the amount of oxalate in plants.

Although oxalate has no known function in animals, it is believed to help plants dispose of calcium. Animals have kidneys that excrete excess calcium. Plants do not. The theory is that the oxalate binds to the excess calcium (much as it does in the human intestine), trapping it in the leaves, bark, and skin. As older leaves are shed, the plant disposes of unwanted calcium. As the plant gets older, the oxalate content tends to increase.

3. *The bioavailability of oxalate differs in foods.* Strawberries and spinach are both high-oxalate foods. However, when people ate equivalent amounts of oxalate in these two foods in tests, those eating spinach had a much greater increase in urinary oxalate. This is because the oxalate in spinach is more bioavailable, or easily absorbed by the body, than it is in strawberries.

If oxalate is present as oxalic acid (the form found in younger plants), it is more bioavailable. If it is present in food as a calcium oxalate salt (the form found in older plants), it is less bioavailable in the intestines and absorption decreases.

Consequently, any food tables that list oxalate values are estimates, and they may well change over time. For those people who must control dietary oxalate, we stress the avoidance of certain foods that have been demonstrated to have consistently higher oxalate levels than others.

Key Issues in Oxalate Control

Controlling your dietary oxalate is not simply a matter of avoiding certain foods. The following are other considerations.

Portion Size

The most important aspect of oxalate control is portion size. For example, the sprig of parsley on your plate may not make a big difference, but if you eat a bowl of the fried parsley favored in some cuisines you have a problem. A piece of squash may not make a difference, but a bowl of acorn squash soup can mean trouble. A few raspberries or strawberries is not the same as a few tablespoons of raspberry or strawberry jam.

If a food with "some" oxalate in it is distilled or concentrated into a sauce or jam, it is likely to have much more oxalate (e.g., tomatoes vs. tomato sauce, strawberries vs. strawberry jam, weak tea vs. strong tea). This is why we caution tea lovers to "brew it weak."

Fat Intake

In people prone to the overabsorption of oxalate, a high-fat diet will cause more oxalate to be absorbed. (See "Fat Malabsorption" in Chapter 9.)

Avoid Vitamin C Supplements

In some people, megadoses of vitamin C above 1000 milligrams per day can be converted to oxalate in the body.

Watch for Hidden Oxalates

Many high-oxalate foods are invisible to the eye. A classic example is the peanut oil used to cook most Chinese food. (Also see Chapters

18 and 21.) Ground nuts are incorporated in all types of recipes, such as pesto sauce made from pine nuts. Pepper may be a heavy seasoning for some at every meal. If oxalate is one of your chief trouble-makers, you must learn which foods are very high in oxalates and where they are found as hidden ingredients.

Oxalates and Seasonal Foods

People with oxalate restrictions on their diets should follow the oxalate chart in the Appendix outlining low-, moderate-, and high-oxalate foods. Many high-oxalate foods are seasonal, which may also help you to remember them.

Winter

Winter means flu season, which causes some people to take megadoses of vitamin C. It is also a time of heavy meals and soups with high-oxalate ingredients. The Thanksgiving to New Year's holiday season is also an oxalate trap. Christmas fruitcake has enough hidden oxalates to seed a stone by New Year's. Foods to watch include

Cranberry sauce
Gumbo soup
Cocoa and/or Ovaltine
Kale and collard greens
Holiday pies made with pecans, pumpkins, or cranberries
Sweet potatoes
Baked beans
Chocolates

Spring

Spring is the season to "get into shape for summer," and that often means large salads and dehydrating exercise regimes. June weddings and seasonal foods contribute to oxalate overload. Foods to watch include

Spinach
Watercress
Draft beer (St. Patrick's Day celebrations)
Leeks

Large quantities of salad
Rhubarb
Sorrel

Summer

More kidney stones are formed in summer than any other season. The combined effects of high-oxalate summer fruits and vegetables with heat, UV sun exposure, and dehydration contribute to this statistic. Foods to watch include

Summer fruits (blackberries, blueberries, raspberries, strawberries)
Green pepper
Summer squash
Some home-canned fruits and jellies
Purple grapes
Iced tea

Fall

Fall is also a high stone-forming season. High-oxalate ingredients are found in many holiday recipes. Foods to control include

Pumpkin
Nuts
Sweet potatoes
Lemon, lime, and orange peel
Fruitcake
Hot tea and cocoa
Cider drinks

Of course, with modern transportation, many so-called seasonal foods are available year-round. Pumpkins may only appear only in the fall, but spinach is found in all four seasons.

All stone formers need to be aware of the oxalate content of foods, but anyone prone to overabsorb oxalate or whose stone formation began with a dietary increase in oxalate must be especially vigilant. Remember, it is not just the specific food but the portion size and the way it is prepared that matter. The classic example is a slice of tomato versus a half cup of tomato sauce.

Finally, when you know you have overindulged, drink two large glasses of water—or more.

18

MODIFYING RECIPES AND CONTROLLING PORTIONS

If there's two cookies or there's ten cookies, before I go to bed, they'll be gone.

For many people, dieting means not being able to eat the things they really enjoy. Therefore, it is important to incorporate the Master Plan into your everyday recipes if you are going to make the long-term changes necessary to control your stone disease. You will see that simple modifications can make a big difference in the oxalate, salt, and protein content of a recipe.

Recipe Modifications

The following guidelines cover key areas in the average diet and will help you to modify your own favorite or family recipes.

Salads

For the stone former, salad ingredients must be carefully selected. Green salads are universally popular, but many of these leafy vegetables contain high amounts of oxalate. On the other hand, fresh vegetables contain a high moisture content and indirectly add water to your diet. You do not have to omit the salad course, for a wide variety of choices are available in the market.

136

Choose:	Instead of:
Lettuce	Escarole
Leaf	Chicory
Boston or butterhead	Dandelion greens
Bibb	Sorrel
Iceberg	Spinach
Simpson	Arugula
Belgium or French endive	Watercress
Cabbage (white)	Chinese cabbage (bok choy)
Radishes	Parsley
Mushrooms	Green peppers
Onions	Celery
Avocado	Chives
Cauliflower	Mustard greens
Oil and vinegar dressing	Commercial dressings (high in salt)

Soups

Soup is often the starter for a full course meal or, in some cases, the meal itself. It can be hearty and thick or light and thin. Most often, except for creamed soups, water is the most plentiful ingredient; therefore, soups make a good choice for the stone former as long as all the other ingredients follow recommended guidelines.

• *Salt.* Canned or convenience soups are notorious for their very high sodium content (1000 mg or more in a serving; see the Appendix, Table 4). Healthy soups can now be found with a lower salt content. Homemade soup is usually far less salty than any soup you can buy in a can. Make sure you cut the amount of salt used in half for the stone former or eliminate it entirely if your palate allows.

• *Oxalate.* Parsley in soup contributes flavor and should be strained out of the broth before serving. Consult the oxalate table in the Appendix when making a favorite soup; okra, spinach, and escarole should be avoided. Gumbos, borscht, and heavy bean soups are an oxalate trap.

• *Calcium.* Creamed soups are made with milk products, which may be a consideration for some stone formers watching their calcium intake. Potatoes or rice put through a blender will "cream" a soup without the addition of milk.

Casseroles and Stews

Mixed dishes or casseroles are excellent choices for the stone former with some minor alterations to classic preparation. The protein ingredients (i.e., fish, chicken, pork, or beef) can be used in smaller amounts, while other ingredients including rice, noodles, or potatoes can extend the dish and contribute no oxalates. The traditional vegetables used in stews such as mushrooms, peas, and onions are low in oxalates. Other vegetables used to layer casseroles must be watched more closely.

Stews give us a good example of how to modify a recipe. Many homes have their favorite beef, veal, or lamb stew. The following steps also modify chicken dishes.

1. Extend the amount of servings. If your recipe feeds four, extend the protein with pasta, rice, potatoes, onions, and carrots so that the recipe feeds six. This addition automatically cuts down on the amount of protein served each person.
2. Substitute low- and moderate-oxalate vegetables for the troublemakers. Cut the amount of salt used in half and substitute a bay leaf or thyme for flavor.
3. Do not sprinkle with parsley or an extra ladle of gravy before serving the stone former.

Sauces and Stocks

Most sauces are a concentration of ingredients. Stock is made by reducing several cups of liquid to one in order to intensify the flavor of the ingredients. This also intensifies the delivery of oxalate and purines to your kidneys. The salt load is increased as well during stock or gravy reduction. Cream in a sauce is less of a problem than the stock base to which it is added.

Since many sauces cannot be made without key ingredients (tomato sauce is not the same without tomatoes), the best advice is to limit the servings of oxalate- and purine-rich sauces and gravies for the stone former. This limitation includes tomato sauce and all gravies made from a stock of meat bones or innards (remember, fish and chicken are meat).

If sauces are added to a casserole—lasagna is a good example— try to add low-oxalate vegetables or more pasta to extend the dish and lower the sauce load in each portion.

Purées are often used as sauce accompaniments for main dishes as well as cakes. These purées should be made with low-oxalate fruits and vegetables. Raspberry and strawberry coulis are not for stone formers.

Cheese and Egg Dishes

Cheese is high in calcium, protein, and salt. Whole eggs are an excellent source of protein. In combination, the portion size of servings in this category is as important as the preparation of these dishes.

Stone formers who eat omelets/eggs and quiches regularly must remember to add up their protein allotment (see the Appendix, Tables 5 and 6) and eliminate high-oxalate vegetables and salt from the preparation. For example, spinach is a favorite in many omelets and cheese pies or quiches. Substitute mushrooms, onions, or broccoli.

Desserts

Cake and pie recipes often call for ingredients that stone formers must avoid. Watch for recipes that call for lemon or orange peel as an ingredient. This is often the case with sponge cakes, layer cakes, and dessert "breads" such as zucchini or carrot cake. A drop of lemon extract may do the flavor trick.

Avoid layering cakes with large amounts of strawberry or raspberry jam or marmalade. Substitute plum, peach, or apple jelly. Frostings should be made with lemon or orange extract rather than the peel of these fruits and not dusted with nuts.

Many cookies are made from ground almonds or pecans. These should be avoided, as well as other desserts made with ground nuts. Flourless chocolate cakes are often made with ground nut "flour." Some recipes call for only a small amount of nuts, which is a possible indulgence if the portions are small. Do not sprinkle extra nuts on top for decoration.

Fruit pies should be made with low- or moderate-oxalate fruits. (See the Appendix, Table 2.)

Chocolate is chocolate. There is really no substitute for this high-oxalate food. Either avoid making chocolate desserts or have the stone former indulge in a few mouthfuls instead of a portion. Cocoa is chocolate and the same restrictions apply.

Portion Control

We have consistently emphasized that *how much* is as important as *what* you are eating. (See also Chapters 8 and 14.) You can eliminate troublemakers from your home recipes and still run into difficulty because of the size of servings.

It is helpful to look at the food on your plate differently. Serve your dinner meal on a smaller size plate. Take a smaller helping of meat and fill the plate with other items such as pasta, rice, potato, or lower-oxalate vegetables and fruits. The meat portion should be considered an accompaniment to the starch and vegetable servings rather than the focal point.

Questions to Ask Yourself

How often do you eat a plateful of food that is heaped to the edges? How big is the piece of meat on that plate? Do you go back for seconds? Thirds? Do you eat leftovers as a late-night snack?

19

HEALTH-FOOD STORE HAZARDS

I've never even seen some of these high-oxalate foods. What's a beet root?

The shelves of a health-food store are stocked with land mines for the stone former. Many otherwise healthy foods are extremely high in oxalates. (See Chapters 8 and 17.) Roots, parsley, and spinach are often the hidden ingredient in a powder or pill base.

For those of you who favor "natural" or vegetarian foods and supplements, a guided tour through the ingredients found in a health-food store is in order. Keep one thing in mind: *Read the label.* Manufacturers must list ingredients in descending order of predominance on the label—by weight, from most to least. Therefore, if you see a high-oxalate food listed first on the label, it is the main ingredient of the product.

The actual oxalate content is rarely reported in the list of ingredients. Any leaf, root, or berry extract can contain a very large amount of oxalate. We have seen many patients whose stone formation dates from the use of a food supplement.

Supplements

Most people do not need to supplement a balanced diet to attain nutritional well-being. This simple fact is often overlooked in the effort to be healthier. For the stone former, supplements should be taken under the advice of a doctor. The addition of certain nutrients in unnatural proportions (as in a megadose of certain vitamins), and not in a food, can actually be the cause of some kidney stones. (See Chapter 8.)

Bases

Most supplements are contained in a "base," and many vitamins, minerals, and powder supplements contain high-oxalate foods in these bases. Making the situation for the stone former even worse, in many cases this high-oxalate base is actually the main ingredient.

Parsley, while very high in oxalate, is an herb that is used only as a garnish in most cuisines. However, health-food products use it frequently as a constituent in their formulas. You will also often find spinach as a base ingredient.

You can find fruit bases as well in certain supplements, such as those consisting of concentrated raspberry, strawberry, orange, bilberry, and grape skin.

If you have been consuming megadoses of supplements with these ingredients in the base, you may be unknowingly increasing your oxalate load.

Garlic Supplements

Garlic tablets have been gaining in popularity. They are now being touted as an excellent way to ward off cancer and improve blood cholesterol levels. Garlic's strong odor is often masked with parsley, which is known for its breath-freshening power. You may get an unsuspecting dose of oxalates with some of these supplements:

- *Natural Brand Garlic and Parsley*—garlic, parsley, and wheat germ oil: avoid
- *Natural Brand Super Garlic*—garlic and soybean oil: avoid
- *Natural Brand Coated Garlic Tablets*—100 milligrams of concentrated garlic
- *Garlique*—garlic, cellulose, and stearic acid
- *Nature's Way Galicin Odor Free*—high-potency garlic powder

Since very little hard data exist on the actual amount of oxalate in food supplements, we generally advise stone formers to avoid these types of products entirely. If an individual feels strongly that a given product is advantageous, we recommend using very little of it.

Muscle-Building Protein Supplements

Health-food stores devote a great deal of shelf space to protein powders. Most of them are very expensive and unnecessary for most healthy adults. It is thought, erroneously, that protein supplements will "build" muscle. For those people who actually have a greater need for protein in their diets, inexpensive and more natural sources of protein such as egg whites and skim milk powder (added to regular milk or mashed potatoes) are recommended.

Protein powders are contraindicated for the stone former, especially uric acid stone formers. Protein requirements for most Americans range from a total of 40 to 100 grams a day. This is an amount easily consumed and too often overconsumed. (See Chapters 14 and 15 on protein.)

Protein supplements can come in a variety of flavors. Chocolate and strawberry are two favorites that contain oxalates. Beware of the double whammy: excessive protein and oxalate-containing flavorings. This dietary overload, coupled with the strenuous physical activity that body builders engage in and the resulting fluid losses, can be the perfect environment for a stone to form.

Herbal Teas

Health-food stores stock herbal teas in every imaginable flavor. Herbal teas often have a lower oxalate content than regular tea. A recent study of herbal teas, which included popular brand names such as Sleepytime and I Love Lemon, contained low levels of oxalates. But you should avoid herbal teas made from foods known to contain high oxalates, as well as those made from other exotic (and questionable) sources.

Some ingredients that are not consumed as a "food" in the American diet have never been analyzed for oxalate. But, because they are from the bark of trees, it is possible that they are high in oxalate and you would therefore be wise to avoid them. For example, uva ursi is a bittersweet berry from a northern-growing evergreen shrub that falls in this category. Others are goldenseal root, ginseng root, sarsaparilla root, yucca, and yellow dock root.

Natural Weight-Loss Regimes

Weight loss plans found in the health-food store often contain roots, berries, seeds, and minerals that have high oxalate levels. Parsley and spearmint are often used as flavoring agents. For example:

- *Herbal Plus, All-Natural Water Pill Herbs* is a natural diuretic—something the kidney stone former does *not* need. It will lead to fluid loss, not sustained weight loss, and it can potentially contribute to stone formation.
- *Ultra Lean Herbal Weight-Loss Plan* incorporates brindel berry and caffeine, which is a diuretic. Avoid this.

Hair Regrowth

Although there is no scientific documentation that any supplement can indeed grow hair, skin, and nails, many products on the market make these claims. The stone former should be cautious of these products, especially those that contain the amino acids that are protein components. This includes L-cysteine, L-methionine, L-glutathione, and gelatin. Following the label instructions to take four or more tablets daily adds unwanted and unhealthy amino acids. Examples of these products include

- *Hair Fitness*—L-cysteine, L-methionine, and amino acids
- *Kal Hair Force*—L-cysteine, L-methionine, L-glutathione, and vitamins

Beverages

If you suffer from lactose intolerance, an inability to digest milk sugar, or an allergy to cow's milk, you must be careful of your choice of milk substitutes.

- *Eden Soy*—a soy milk beverage that contains oxalates
- *Eden Rice Beverage*—a better choice with no oxalates

For those stone formers trying to break a caffeine habit by replacing coffee with a "healthy" beverage, do *not* try Cafix. Cafix is made of malt, chicory, barley, and beet root. An instant beverage, like Postum (made from cereal grains), would be preferable.

Vegetarian Burgers

If you are replacing meat in your diet for philosophical or health reasons, the many vegetarian burgers on the market may seem like a healthy alternative. But not all vegetarian burgers are created alike. Stone formers must be alert to the total protein in their diet and soy is still a source of protein. Also, tofu, which is fermented soy milk made into a curd, is listed as a high-oxalate food. Following are some of the popular options for vegetarian burgers:

- *Nature's Burger* is made of barley, brown rice, oats, and wheat. It has soy as the least ingredient.
- *VejaLinks, RediBurgers, and Big Franks* all have vegetable protein, wheat gluten, and soy as ingredients. One Big Frank provides 7 grams of protein.
- *Tofu burgers* are toasted brown rice flour, cornmeal, and soy.

Switching to a vegetarian diet is not the answer to curing kidney stones. Vegetarianism will most likely lower your total protein and fat intake but may add more oxalates to your diet. Balancing all the different food groups is very important.

Laxatives

Laxative overuse can create its own special type of stone-forming process. (See Chapter 10.) Following are some of the laxatives that can be found at health-food stores:

- *Colon Cleaner*—ingredients include wheat grass and buckhorn (of unknown but questionable oxalate content), rhubarb

(high in oxalates), and whey (milk protein, which should be limited)
- *Herbal Laxative*—ingredients include questionable herbs like senna and buckhorn bark
- *Psyllium*—a safe laxative because it consists of soluble fiber and does not contain significant amounts of oxalate.

Some diuretics contain parsley, which should be avoided.

Energy Bars

These replacements for candy bars are high in protein and often have nuts and chocolate as ingredients. Avoid these choices and keep in mind other alternatives such as:

- *Power Bar*—one apple cinnamon bar has 10 grams of protein
- *Tiger Sport*—comes in vanilla or carob, 6 grams of protein provided

Keep a mental count of the amount of protein grams you consume daily. These bars provide about one meal's worth of protein.

The Juice Craze

Juices are in vogue. Various vegetable and fruit juices are bottled and enticingly displayed. Mixed varieties are especially popular, such as cran-lemonade or orange-pineapple. But some juices contain superconcentrated amounts of oxalates:

Vegetable juices—made from tomatoes, carrots, celery roots, beet roots, lactic acid, and sea salt
Beet root juice
Carrot juice
Celery root juice
Cranberry juice

Instead, choose:

Apple juice
Mango nectar
Potato juice

Pastas

There are hundreds of shapes, sizes, thicknesses, and colors of pasta in the health-food store—as well as at your local supermarket. Pastas should definitely be incorporated in your diet. But try to avoid the tricolor vegetable pastas that contain spinach, beet, or tomato juice. The plain and simple pastas are the best choices.

Candies and Cookies

If you crave a chocolate substitute, you might want to try a carob bar. Although high in fat, as long as it does not have nuts or chocolate, it is an acceptable alternative.

Apple cinnamon and carob chip cookies without nuts are also good choices.

The newest breath fresheners on the market are pills of distilled parsley—"nature's breath freshener." Parsley is a high-oxalate food, even more so in its distilled form. After you ingest a pack of these, we can assure you that your breath will be much better, but your kidneys won't.

Read Labels in the Health-Food Store

There are many items in the health-food store that are just that— natural and basically healthy. But stone formers have specific and different guidelines they must follow. *Read label ingredients carefully* before you purchase and ingest any food or supplement. The health-food store is often an oxalate trap.

20

SPECIAL OCCASIONS

Parties and Other Excuses to Cheat

You have to go to these parties and you get stuck eating everything the doctor told you not to eat.

Holidays are like the weekends—it's my time to cheat.

People tend to overindulge on special occasions and use them as an excuse to ignore their diets. Parties, weddings, and holiday meals often begin with lengthy cocktail hours, which can lead to a breakdown in inhibitions that extends into the dining room. Large portions and second helpings of foods with high-oxalate, salt, and protein content can lead to trouble for the stone former. You must learn to skate around the thin ice at the holiday and buffet table and wash down large meals with plenty of water or healthy fluids.

The following is a guide to various special-occasion menus. It is designed to help you identify and avoid troublemakers and find substitutes at large buffets and multicourse meals.

Thanksgiving

Many people consider the period between Thanksgiving and New Year's "the season to be merry," which translates into cheating on their diets and indulging in otherwise forbidden foods. Holiday partying and bingeing and high-oxalate foods like pumpkins, sweet potatoes, and nuts, which are part of many recipes, make this a high-stone-forming season. The boxes of chocolates that appear on co-workers' desks and as house presents are particularly risky.

The following two Thanksgiving menus outline two different approaches to this popular holiday meal.

Thanksgiving Dinner to Watch Out For

Hors d'Oeuvres

1 ounce salted peanuts — A handful of salted peanuts will fulfill your daily oxalate intake and add unwanted salt before you even sit down to dinner.

1 stalk celery — An innocuous "diet" food for most, celery is a moderate source of oxalate and salt for the stone former.

2 six-ounce glasses rosé wine — Watch your alcohol, which leads to dehydration, and opt instead for healthy fluids to dilute the feast to come.

Appetizer

1 cup leek soup — Autumnal soup ingredients like leeks, spinach, and watercress eat up your oxalate allowance; soups are also high in salt.

Main Course

10 ounces roast turkey— white and dark meat — Limit animal protein to a 3-ounce meat serving about the size of a deck of cards. If you overindulge (it *is* Thanksgiving), drink lots of water.

2 ounces gravy — Gravy increases uric acid, a culprit in stone formation.

3 ounces chestnut stuffing — Grandma's stuffing may also be filled with celery and parsley—high in oxalates—and should be avoided by the stone former. Avoid sausage in stuffing, which adds unwanted protein.

1 baked sweet potato — An oxalate-rich root vegetable.

$^1/_2$ cup spinach

A vegetable with one of the highest concentrations of oxalate. Omit it from your diet.

$^1/_2$ cup green beans

Another medium source of oxalate; don't have a lot of it. Better choices include broccoli, cauliflower, peas, and turnips.

2 ounces cranberry sauce

Beware of berries, many contain oxalate, including cranberries. A cranberry-orange relish would be even worse due to the oxalate-rich orange peel. Fruit sauces prepared from apples, apricots, or mangoes offer satisfying alternatives.

1 cracked wheat roll

Don't be fooled by this seemingly healthy choice; wheat germ is a land mine of oxalate. Limit yourself to one if you don't know the ingredients.

Dessert

1 slice pecan pie

Pecans provide a superrich source of oxalates, as do pumpkin and rhubarb. As a conclusion to this meal, this dessert means you are no longer treading water but are officially over your head in oxalate.

2 cups (2 oz) tea

Tea and cocoa are higher in oxalate than coffee. Try silver tea instead— hot water with a drop of lemon juice.

Assorted chocolates

Chocolate-covered nuts are doubly dangerous.

After-dinner drink

The key word is *moderation*. If you have had alcohol with dinner, this is a good time to stop. Make a habit of ending any and every large meal with a 12-ounce glass of water.

Thanksgiving Dinner to Be Grateful For

Hors d'Oeuvres

Raw vegetable platter: cauliflower, broccoli, radishes, mushrooms	Low in oxalates and high in complex carbohydrates, this is a filling combo to start with.
4-ounce white wine spritzer	Lighter and less dehydrating than other cocktails.

Appetizer

Potato-and-turnip soup	Potato-based soups are better choices, but the sodium level is still high. Avoid the parsley garnish.

Main Course

3 ounces roast turkey	Limit the serving size and gravy. Fill your plate with other healthy choices.
$1/2$ cup bread stuffing	White bread is preferable to whole wheat; recipes for rice stuffings with onions and mushrooms are also fine.
$1/2$ cup mashed potatoes with milk	White potatoes are oxalate-free; enjoy extra helpings of this complex carbohydrate.
$1/2$ cup brussels sprouts	Other acceptable choices include broccoli and cabbage.
$1/2$ cup carrots	Watch out for serving size.
$1/2$ cup turnips	
$1/2$ cup creamed onions	A traditional Thanksgiving dish that you can indulge in.
$1/2$ cup applesauce	Good choice for a side dish or dessert.
2 dinner rolls	Rolls from white flour provide the least amount of oxalate.

Dessert

1 slice cherry, peach, or apple pie	Apple pie is the best choice of the usual Thanksgiving fare.
Sorbet or fruit ice	Clears the palate and the kidneys.
Water or healthy fluids throughout the meal	

If you have overindulged despite your good intentions and the warnings in this menu, be sure to drink two 12-ounces glasses of water before bedtime.

If you consume large amounts of high-oxalate or salty foods in one meal and combine them with large amounts of protein and alcohol, you risk oversaturating your urine with stone-forming elements. An immediate balancing act is in order:

- Drink copious amounts of water or healthy fluids during and after the meal and the following day.
- Go back to a strict limited-oxalate and protein diet.
- Cut back on salt.

Thanksgiving dinner can be an enjoyable and healthful meal. Remember, your kidneys must now prepare to face Christmas parties and further holiday festivities.

Barbecue

Although barbecue is enjoyed year-round, summer is traditionally barbecue season. A barbecue is an occasion with a number of potential troublemakers.

Barbecue—The Bad

Chips and dips	Potato chips and pretzels are very salty, and the dip adds extra fat.
A pitcher of draft beer	Poor choice; it is loaded with oxalates, and alcohol is especially dehydrating on a hot summer day.
A side of barbecued ribs	High in salt and too much protein and fat.
Grilled vegetables	Tomatoes, eggplants, and green peppers look great on the plate, but all contain oxalates.

Spinach salad	Spinach is at the top of the taboo list of oxalate-rich food. Bacon bits are salty.
Iced tea	In the top ten foods high in oxalates.
Brownies with walnuts	Chocolate and nuts are highest in oxalates.
Fresh strawberries	More unwanted oxalates you had best avoid.

Barbecue—The Good

16 ounces lemonade	Lemonade *without* the lemon rind is a healthy choice. Fill the glass with ice for more water.
Marinated chicken breast	A growing favorite on barbecue menus, it is a great choice and portion-controlled, since chicken breasts are usually 4 to 6 ounces raw. Eat just one. Watch out for ingredients in the marinade like soy sauce.
Hamburger or hot dog	One of either.
Baked Idaho potato	Good choice.
1/2 cup cole slaw	Raw cabbage and carrots dressed with mayonnaise, a little vinegar, and sugar is a fine side dish.
1 ear corn on the cob	An ear of summer corn with a little butter is fine.
Lettuce salad	Iceberg lettuce, a wedge of fresh beefsteak tomatoes (some oxalates here), and onion with oil and vinegar is also allowed.
1 wedge watermelon	Sweet and delicious, this fruit is full of water.
Roasted marshmallows	A traditional end to a barbecue—marshmallows are sugar and starch and contain no oxalates.

Wedding Banquet

Members of the wedding party will diet for several months before the event in order to fit into their dresses and tuxedoes, but on that special day, anything goes.

While it seems unfair to have to watch what you are eating on this particular occasion, there are certain tidbits that can cause a great deal of trouble.

Wedding Banquet—The Bad

Beverage

Champagne	Unlimited amounts cause dehydration.

Hors d'Oeuvres

Caviar on wheat thins Sweetbreads in puff pastry Chidren livers wrapped in bacon	These tempting morsels contain purines—dangerous for the uric acid stone former.

Appetizer

Watercress soup	This kind of soup is high in oxalates and possibly sodium.

Main Course

Prime rib au jus	Traditionally prime rib is served as a large portion—ask for a half serving when placing your order.
Sweet potato croquettes	This is another oxalate-containing root vegetable.
Green bean salad with walnut dressing	Green beans, a moderate oxalate-containing item, are okay alone, but the addition of nuts pushes the limit on oxalates.

Dessert

Orange almond wedding cake	Orange rind and almonds—high-oxalate ingredients—lurk within this elegant-looking cake.

Chocolate-covered strawberries Tea	A double dose of oxalates, this is definitely not the right choice to end the meal.

Wedding Banquet—The Good

Beverage

Champagne	Make a toast and enjoy *one* glass.
Mineral water	Water is always available at a wed-
Ice Water	ding dinner—indulge yourself.

Hors d'Oeuvres

Scotch salmon with dill butter on white toast points Stuffed mushrooms Tomatoes stuffed with crabmeat Shrimp cocktail	All these appetizers have acceptable oxalate content.

Appetizer

Mixed iceberg lettuce salad with vinaigrette dressing	This is a very safe standard salad for the stone former.

Main Course

Stuffed breast of veal	Stuffed with white bread, garlic, and herbs, this is a safe choice.
Wild rice pilaf Rissole potatoes	Good choices.
Buttered fancy french peas	This is a low-oxalate veggie.

Dessert

Wedding white cake with Grand Marnier buttercream icing	Traditional wedding cakes are often simple, elegant, and safe for the stone former.
Coffee	Good choice
Ice water	Drinking water at the end of every big meal is a healthy habit to develop.

Breakfast Buffet

Many parties, weddings, and weekend occasions start or end with a breakfast buffet. Many hotels and restaurants offer this type of meal in place of sit-down service for Sunday brunch. The tips on the following menu can also guide the business traveler ordering from room service in the morning.

Breakfast Buffet—The Bad

Cranberry juice	This has moderate oxalates.
Corn muffins, Bran muffins, Blueberry muffins	There are moderate oxalates in cornmeal, bran, and added berries.
Strawberry jam, Orange marmalade	These toppings have concentrated oxalates.
Fruited yogurt	Avoid the high-oxalate fruit yogurts like strawberry and raspberry.
Bacon strips, Sausage links	These combine protein, fat, and salt.
Western omelet, Spanish omelet	Avoid eggs with ingredients containing oxalates like green peppers and tomatoes.
Figs, Fresh strawberries	These fruits are high in oxalates.
Hot Cocoa, Ovaltine, Tea	These beverages contain oxalates.

Breakfast Buffet—The Good

Orange juice, Grapefruit juice, Pineapple juice	These juices are low in oxalates, and you can always add water or ice for extra fluid.
Bagels, English muffins, Assorted rolls	All these bread choices are made from white flour and are low in oxalates.
Butter, Honey, Margarine, Apple butter	These spreads are low in oxalates, but don't go overboard with butter and margarine.
Scrambled eggs, Shirred eggs, American cheese omelet	Watch your protein with eggs and dairy.

Vanilla, lemon, or coffee yogurt	Flavored yogurts are a better choice than fruited ones.
Waffles, Pancakes, French toast	These are best if made with white flour.
Pancake syrup	Sugar is safe.
Banana, Melon wedges	The riper the fruit, the lower the oxalate content.
Low-fat milk	Be sure to consume the prescribed two servings of dairy every day; low-fat is best.

Four Pitfalls of Special Occasions

There are four basic pitfalls the stone former must avoid while enjoying holiday or party fare:

1. *Protein Gluttony.* Tidbits combine with large amounts of red and white meat to send your uric acid levels soaring.
2. *Oxalate Overload.* The garnishes, hidden ingredients, and seasonal fruits and vegetables can add up to extremely high oxalate consumption that is way beyond your daily or weekly levels.
3. *Alcohol Overload.* Alcohol dehydrates you *and* can diminish your inhibitions and good intentions regarding your diet. That is a potent combination.
4. *Overeating.* It is all too easy to eat too much. Between second portions at buffets and four- to six-course meals, your kidneys must process an enormous load of waste products. If the celebrations go on for several days or, in the case of the holiday season, several months, these wastes can seed a stone.

21

ETHNIC CUISINES

The hardest part is arguing in a restaurant in front of the waiter—saying you can't have that . . . and I become the nagging wife. I just don't trust him on his own.

I'm out with a customer who, unfortunately, ordered lamb chops as big as my head. What was I supposed to do— pick at a salad?

We go to McDonald's a lot with the kids. I try to eat the salad—I'll steal the kids' fries. But the chicken is weird in the salad—nothing lived that is shaped like that. So I cover it in dressing.

Restaurant menus are full of temptations for the stone former. Making the matter worse, your favorite dish or cuisine may contain hidden troublemakers. Knowing which foods to avoid before going into a restaurant can help you eliminate many dietary slips.

The advice in this chapter will help you choose dishes from many types of cuisines. It will also serve as a convenient guide if you are vacationing in the country of origin or regularly make certain ethnic dishes.

Chinese

I eat Chinese food religiously once a week.

The Chinese are known for their healthful eating habits: stir-fried vegetables, steamed fish, lots of rice, and tea. For the stone former, though, there are hidden ingredients that must be carefully avoided. These include

1. Peanut oil, which is used to cook most dishes and which is high in oxalates
2. Vegetables like bok choy, which are high in oxalates and found in chow mein and many other dishes
3. Salt in the form of soy sauce and MSG (monosodium glutamate), which is a common seasoning used to prepare many dishes.
4. Soybeans, which are used to create a wide variety of products, from tofu (bean curd, black bean sauce) to soy sauces. This excellent source of protein is unfortunately high in oxalates.

On the other hand, there are many excellent choices available if you know how to order.

Appetizers

Many appetizers are deep-fried in peanut oil, which should be avoided. Fried food is not inherently bad for stone formers, but peanut oil is because of its oxalate content. Peanut oil is valued for frying because of its high "smoke point." It is high in monounsaturated and polyunsaturated fats.

Avoid   spareribs (high in protein, fat, and sodium)

Good Choice   steamed dumplings, paper-wrapped chicken

Soup

All soups are salty. Offset this by drinking lots of water and don't overindulge in soy sauce later in the meal.

Avoid   bean curd with vegetables (oxalates in bean curd), egg drop soup (egg adds excess protein)

Good Choice   wonton soup, sizzling rice soup, minced chicken corn soup

Poultry

Avoid   chicken with cashews

Special Order   white-meat chicken with mixed vegetables (eliminate spinach or bok choy)

Good Choice   chicken and broccoli, chicken with snow peas

Seafood

Avoid   lobster in black bean sauce

Special Order   shrimp with mixed vegetables, shrimp with lobster sauce (eggs in sauce add protein; watch portions on this)

Good Choice   lobster in shell, shrimp and broccoli with garlic sauce, scallops in hot and spicy sauce

Pork

Avoid   pork in hot sauce with peanuts

Special Order   roast pork with mixed vegetables

Better Choice   pork with scallions, moo shu pork with pancakes

Beef

Avoid   beef with hot sauce and peanuts

Good Choice   beef with snow peas, beef with scallions

Vegetables

Avoid   bean curd home-style

Special Order   mixed vegetables (avoid bok choy and spinach)

Acceptable Choice   sautéed hot and spicy string beans (watch what oil is used)

Rice and Noodles

Avoid   subgum fried rice, fried rice

Great Choice   lo mein (chicken, pork, beef, vegetable, or shrimp), steamed rice

Desserts

Avoid pistachio and chocolate ice cream (choose vanilla)

Good Choice orange quarters, pineapple slices, fortune cookie, litchi nuts (litchi is a fruit, not a nut)

Beverages

Avoid tea, Chinese beer (high in sodium)

Mexican

Mexican food has received some bad press recently regarding its high fat content. This is not necessarily true and can be avoided. Mole (meaning "concoction") sauce, commonly served with poultry, is a deep reddish-brown sauce made from a blend of onion, garlic, several chili peppers, ground seeds (such as sesame or pumpkin), and a small amount of Mexican chocolate. This oxalate-containing food should be avoided. The three main problem areas for the stone former eating Mexican food are:

- Salt
- Protein
- Oxalate and purine content of certain foods such as beans

Appetizers

Avoid salsa (chilies, cilantro, Mexican parsley), nachos, nachos with chorizos, chalupas (cheese and meat are excessive), quesadillas

Good Choice gambas al ajilo (sautéed garlic shrimp), guacamole, ceviche (avoid cilantro on top)

Soup

Avoid black bean soup

Better Choice gazpacho, Spanish mixed salad (avoid any parsley or cilantro)

Mexican Entrées

Avoid   chimichanga (deep-fried tortilla stuffed with beef), pollo mole poblano (chicken served with spicy mole sauce), burritos with refried beans and cheese

Good Choice   entrecot manana (limit serving to 4 oz), pollo al ajilo, seafood enchiladas, fajitas (meat, shrimp, or chicken), arroz con pollo, camarones al ajilo (shrimp sautéed in garlic sauce)

Combination Platters

Avoid   tacos, tostada, refried beans

Greek

While meat is at a premium on the small Greek islands, cheese is found in abundance in Greek recipes. Feta cheese—a white, crumbly, salty cheese made from goat's milk—is served in salads and as an ingredient in casseroles and other dishes. When eating Greek food, stone formers must watch for things wrapped in grape leaves and spinach, which are found in many dishes. Most desserts are made with honey and nuts, which are high in oxalates.

Appetizers

Avoid   horta salada (steamed chicory in olive oil), spanakopita (spinach and feta wrapped in dough)

Special Order   Greek salad (leave out the feta and grape leaves, watch very salty olives and anchovies)

Entrées

Avoid   kokoretsi (sweetbreads and hearts), moussaka

Good Choice   (watch portion size): arni souvlas (roast lamb), kontosouvli (marinated roast pork), souvlaki (chicken or lamb kebobs)

Desserts

Avoid   baklava, kataifi

Better Choice   melopitta (honey cheesecake), galacrobourecco (phyllo pastry with custard center)

French

French food is known for its gravies (essence of purine), portion sizes, and the creative and delicious presentation of vegetables such as spinach. All of these delights must be either avoided or taken in moderation by the stone former.

Appetizers

Avoid   paté de foie gras

Special Order   mixed salad (dressing on the side)

Good Choice   fresh asparagus vinaigrette, coquilles Saint-Jacques (scallops in wine sauce)

Soup

Avoid   cream of watercress soup

Better Choice   consommé

Entrées

Avoid   beef Wellington (beef covered with goose liver paté)

Portion Control   steak au poivre

Better Choice (watch for sauces)   poached salmon, baked breast of chicken, bouillabaisse, coq au vin, filet de veau

Vegetables

Avoid   creamed spinach

Good Choice   julienne carrots, petite peas

Desserts

Avoid   profiteroles au chocolat, chocolate mousse

Special Order   sorbet (avoid strawberry or raspberry)

Best Choice   fresh fruit salad (avoid strawberries)

Best Idea   If you must indulge, take a spoon and share

Japanese

The Japanese are known for their healthy, low-fat diet with fish and rice as its base. But not everything in this cuisine is appropriate for the stone former. Soybeans, bean curd or tofu, and miso (soybean paste) are protein sources that are high in oxalates. Soy sauce is pure salt, and the sushi bar is an invitation to eat excess protein, albeit in small bites.

Appetizers

Avoid   ohitashi (spinach in soy sauce), tofu salad with miso dressing

Good Choice   shumai (steamed dumplings), yakitori (broiled chicken on skewers)

Entrées

Avoid   yudofu (cooked, hot tofu), dengaku (grilled tofu with miso)

Watch Salty Sauce   chicken teriyaki, beef teriyaki

Good Choice   soba (noodles), yosenabe (noodles, seafood and vegetables in broth), shumai (steamed seafood dumplings)

Sushi and Sashimi

Beware of the amount of protein consumed in little bites.

Desserts

Avoid   yokan (red bean cake)

Special Order   ice cream (avoid green tea and red bean)

Good Choice   Fresh fruit in season (avoid strawberries)

Beverage

Avoid   green tea

Italian

The cornerstone of Italian food is tomato sauce, which is simply concentrated oxalates. Stone formers must also be careful when ordering dark green vegetables such as arugula salads, which have huge oxalate levels. Most Italian restaurants also serve large portions.

Soup

Avoid   Stracciatella (egg drop soup with Parmesan cheese, spinach, and pasta), tortelloni in brodo (cheese-filled pasta, spinach, tomato, and egg in consommé), minestrone (made with spinach and beans)

Salad

Avoid   escarole and chicory in salads

Special Order   Caesar salad (avoid the anchovies)

Share   arugula and Belgian endive served with vinaigrette

Good Choice   insalata di casa, shrimp cocktail (go lightly on sauce and watch protein portions)

Appetizers

Avoid   antipasto, Spanish peppers, and anchovies

Good Choice   baked clams, steamed clams, or mussels in a white wine sauce (avoid parsley garnish)

Pasta

Avoid   cannelloni (stuffed with spinach, cheese, and tomato), spinach lasagna

Share   manicotti, ziti, fettucini Alfredo

Special Order   tortellini (avoid spinach or cheese), pasta primavera (eliminate spinach or escarole)

Watch Amount of Sauce   spaghetti with tomato sauce, spaghetti with meatballs or sausage

Best Choice   angel hair with white clam sauce, macaroni with broccoli

Entrées

Avoid   eggplant parmigiana

Share   veal and chicken parmigiana

Good Choice (watch portion size)   shrimp primavera, shrimp scampi, veal piccata, chicken marsala

Bread

Share   bruschetta, focaccia

Best Choice   baghetta (sourdough)

Desserts

Avoid   spumoni (ice cream with chocolate and nuts), tortoni (ice cream topped with almonds), cannoli (made with bits of chocolate, candied citron, and nuts)

Special Order   Italian ice (no chocolate), rum cake (avoid nut-encrusted icing)

American

American cuisine is difficult to define, since the United States is such a melting pot of world cuisines. In general, though, generous serving sizes are common as well as generous amounts of salt, sugar, and fat in different combinations.

Appetizers

Avoid   nachos, potato chips, mixed nuts, fried mozzarella sticks, buffalo wings (all salty)

Special Order   potato skins (okay if baked, not fried)

Good Choice   shrimp cocktail

Soup

Avoid   gumbo

Good Choice   chicken noodle

Salad Bars

Avoid   beets, spinach

Portion Control   bacon bits, olives, cheese, tomatoes

Best Choice   lettuce, onions, avocado, mushrooms

Entrée Salads

Avoid   spinach salad

Sandwiches

Avoid   Philadelphia cheese steak, Reuben sandwich (large and salty portions)

Best Choice   grilled chicken breast, roast beef, tuna

Burgers

Avoid   chili burger, bacon cheeseburger

Good Choice   beef hamburger (3 oz serving), turkey burger

Toppings

Safe Choice   sautéed onions, mushrooms, lettuce, jalapeño pepper

Small Amounts   green peppers, tomato, barbecue sauce

Vegetable and Starches

Avoid   collards, kale, creamed spinach

Share   french fries

Good Choice   baked potato, rice, corn on the cob, peas, broccoli

Entrées

Avoid   barbecued beef ribs and chicken (large, salty servings)

Better Choice   shrimp (best when steamed or broiled), broiled fresh fish, grilled chicken, steak (filet mignon); watch all portion sizes

Desserts

Avoid   chocolate cake, hot fudge sundae, mud pie

Special Order   ice cream pies (watch for chocolate, strawberry, nuts), sundaes (watch toppings)

Best Choice   apple pie and sorbet

Indian

The distinctive blending of spices and seasonings makes Indian food so interesting and appealing. This cuisine accentuates vegetables and rice and de-emphasizes protein, a healthy diet for a stone former. But beware of the pulses (beans, chickpeas, and lentils puréed together)

and the spinach found in many recipes or as a side dish. These have high amounts of oxalates. Lastly, beware of foods cooked in coconut milk (oxalates and calcium-containing) and ghee; clarified butter adds excess fat.

Soup

Avoid mulligatawny soup (lightly spiced lentil), coconut soup (coconut and pistachio nuts), poppy seed soup (almond, poppy seed, milk, and coconut cream)

Appetizers

Avoid piazi (onion with fresh lentils), papadum (thin lentil wafers)

Share meat, samosa (minced lamb, peas, onions, and herbs, deep-fried)

Good Choice samosa (potatoes, peas, and herbs), shrimp poori, fish kebab, and mixed green salad

Entrées

Avoid chicken tikka masala (cooked with almonds), beef, lamb, or chicken shag (cooked with spinach)

Better Choice chicken tandoori and lamb, beef, or shrimp kebab

Vegetarian

Avoid bhindi bhaji (okra and onion), mottor or shag ponir (spinach and green peas), chana and shag bhaji (fried spinach), dal (lentils)

Special Order mixed vegetable curry (specify vegetables)

Good Choice aloo mottor gobi (potatoes, green peas, and cauliflower cooked with spices)

Rice Specialties

Special Watch chicken biryani (watch out for almonds), beef or lamb biryani, vegetable biryani (watch for almonds, okra, spinach)

Homemade Breads

Avoid   chapati (whole wheat bread), puris (fried whole wheat bread)

Best Choice   naan (white flat bread)

Condiments

Avoid   dals (lentils, peas, beans, and salt)

Better Choice   mango chutney

Beverages

Avoid   tea

Portion Control   mango lassi (yogurt counts toward your daily calcium allowance)

Desserts

Avoid   kulfi (nuts)

Share   rasmalai (homemade cheese balls in sweet cream)

Good Choice   firni (Indian rice pudding)

22

STAYING MOTIVATED

It's very hard not to eat fried food or fast food in our world.

From my perspective as his wife, there's always a constant struggle. I feel that I have to control what he eats.

If I lose a lot of weight, then I feel that I deserve to go out and eat. So I go out and put on 15 pounds. I'm my own worst enemy.

One week after a kidney stone attack, every person undergoing this excruciating experience vows to do *anything and everything* to avoid another similar episode. Six months later, however, when the pain is a distant memory, many people begin to fall off the wagon. Life is full of temptations. That lasagna and chocolate fudge cake look very appealing, and it is only a "little cheat." One dietary indiscretion is not going to hurt . . . or is it?

The first question you must ask yourself is: "What is my risk level?" If you fall into the high-risk group as defined in Chapter 13, you need to make permanent changes in your routine. If you cannot control your diet and habits, you will be a perennial patient. One or two "indulgences" coupled with warm-weather dehydration and you will be back at the emergency room.

If your risk is moderate, you may be able to allow yourself some latitude. But *some* indulgence does not mean once a day, every day.

If you have had three stone episodes, each following a crash diet, you probably will be fine if you simply avoid this bad practice. You are at low risk for another episode if you stay away from your troublemaker. Unfortunately, once you put on so much extra weight that you need to diet again, you are at much higher risk. Indulgence becomes a yo-yo dieting syndrome.

How Far Can You Deviate?

Every person must realistically assess his or her risk potential. I saw a patient who never made a stone until a friend convinced her that a daily glass of cranberry and grapefruit juice with a teaspoon of vinegar would stop colds and "clean out the system." She began to drink 8 ounces of this mixture every morning before breakfast and again before bed, and one month later she had her first episode of colic. Assuming that there are no other reasons for your stone-forming propensity, you could probably resume most of your old habits as long as you stopped your new acidic cocktail.

On the other hand, if you have *medullary sponge kidney* and have already made a dozen stones, you obviously have much less license to indulge. Follow the four steps of the Master Plan and incorporate the necessary changes into your diet and lifestyle.

Diluting the Mistake

The first rule of overindulgence is to dilute the mistake. If you consider eating lasagna and chocolate cake, which are relatively high in oxalates and full of calories, you know that is not the best meal for your stone problem. But when you are at a party, you cannot refuse dinner if this is what is put on the table. In such a situation, eat what you are served, but don't go back for seconds, and drink lots of fluids. You must be sure to increase your urine flow if you eat a high-oxalate meal. If your profile is a "protein glutton," and you eat 10 ounces of steak (please do not go for 16 ounces), drink several glasses of water during and after the meal. And stay away from iced tea.

The last rule of overindulgence is *remember the pain*.

Kidney stones can be prevented. There are few medical conditions that are as painful—or as easily controlled. They really are "what you eat." Have a sign permanently attached to your refrigerator: No More Kidney Stones!

PART THREE

MEDICINES, SPECIALISTS, AND PROCEDURES

There are some remedies worse than the disease.
—PUBLILIUS SYRUS, MAXIM 301

23

CHOOSING A SPECIALIST

The best doctors in the world are Doctor Diet, Doctor Quiet, and Doctor Merryman.

—Jonathan Swift (1667–1745)

There are a number of medical specialists who treat kidney stone disease. These usually include urologists, nephrologists, endocrinologists, and infectious disease specialists, as well as your primary care physician. It is sometimes confusing as to who does what. The following descriptions explain the medical subspecialties, the procedures they usually handle, and who usually treats the complications of kidney stone disease.

Who Does What

The Internist or Family Practitioner

Your primary care physician may see a few stone episodes in a year. This physician may be quite competent to manage your pain and the passing of a stone with no complicating factors. Nevertheless, the average doctor engaged in primary care is likely to be unfamiliar with the treatment of any complications that can occur.

If you are reading this book, there is a good chance that you have passed more than one stone or have had some trouble beyond a few hours of pain with a stone. Your primary care doctor will probably have referred you to one of the following physicians.

The Urologist

Most people will be referred to a urologist. The urologist first trains as a surgeon and then specializes in the urinary tract. This is the specialist most people with retained stones will visit. The urologist does *cystoscopies* (looks inside your bladder), *catheterization* to relieve urinary obstruction, operates the *lithotripter* (see Chapter 25), and performs any type of surgery necessary to the urinary tract.

Urologists also handle prostate problems, malignancies and other tumors of the urinary tract, testicular problems, voiding problems, and surgical adrenal disease. Some urologists concentrate on surgery and other interventions but prefer to leave stone prevention and the metabolic evaluation of their patients to the medical subspecialists. Others have made metabolic problems their interest and are able to manage stone formers throughout their illness.

The Nephrologist

The nephrologist is first trained in internal medicine and then specializes in the kidney. Some nephrologists are particularly interested in dialysis or renal immunology and have only a limited knowledge about managing stones and urinary tract infections. This is the specialty that is usually called in to manage people who have had stone disease.

I am a nephrologist who did research in an endocrinology laboratory that specialized in calcium metabolism. Therefore, my training and experience cross the boundaries between the specialties of nephrology and endocrinology.

The Endocrinologist

The endocrinologist first trains as an internist and then specializes in metabolism and the regulation of the glandular hormones in the body. This specialist may be called in to handle a person with *hyperparathyroidism* or other metabolic disorders at the heart of a stone problem. Some endocrinologists specialize in thyroid problems, diabetes, or other hormonal problems and have little experience with calcium problems such as kidney stones.

Some physicians from endocrinology and nephrology have an interest in both kidney stones and metabolic bone disease.

Infectious Disease Specialists

The infectious disease physician specializes in bacterial and viral infections. This includes most communicable diseases.

Since urinary infections can complicate stone disease, some infectious disease specialists have expertise in the urinary tract. People with difficult struvite stone disease may require the involvement of an infectious disease specialist.

How Do You Find Out Whom to See?

Most of you will have seen a urologist. Your urologist may be trained and interested in evaluation as well as direct intervention. However, since urologists are initially trained as surgeons, many will refer you to a medical specialist to manage the metabolic evaluation and preventative aspects of your care once you are no longer passing a stone or having trouble with one causing obstruction. You can ask your urologist to make this referral. If this avenue is not available to you, you can call the nearest medical school to see who has a particular interest in stone prevention.

Do not be afraid to ask questions about procedures, medications, and the experience of your doctor. For example, if you have had cystine stones and suffer from the unusual problem of *cystinuria*, you need a nephrologist or endocrinologist who has experience in treating this disease.

If your problem is unusual and you require some type of procedure, do not be afraid to ask about your doctor's experience.

24

MEDICATIONS

A desire to take medicine is a feature which distinguishes men from other animals.

—Sir William Osler

Throughout medical history, people have taken a wild assortment of remedies to cure real and imagined ailments. For centuries, bizarre herbal concoctions have been tried in order to stop the pain of kidney stones and remove them. Medieval medicinal potions claiming to cure "a bad case of gravel" were remarkable more for their inspiration than their effectiveness. One such potion contained

> snail-shells and bees of each an equal quantity . . . dry them in an oven . . . then beat to a very fine powder of which give as much as will lie on a sixpence . . . in bean flower water every morning. . . . This has been found to break the Stone and force a speedy passage of urine. (Robert Bulkeley, 1641)

Many cures for "gravel" were mixed with wine, which may have accounted for their popularity.

This chapter describes the modern medications that are used to treat various kidney stone problems. As you will see, we have come a long way from pulverized bees, but we still rely on natural substances for relief of certain conditions. The descriptions are designed only to give you information about these medications in case they are prescribed by your doctor. When used properly, they can help you control stone disease. *Do not self-medicate or change doses without seeking medical advice. The improper use of medication can hurt you.*

Who Needs to Take Medications

Four out of five people who consult me for stone problems can be managed without any medications. Most people can remain stone-free simply by following the dietary and lifestyle guidelines in this book. Sometimes I will follow a patient for a while with just dietary advice to see if medication is necessary. I am more likely to prescribe medication if there have been multiple stone episodes, difficulty in passing stones, or prior urological intervention, such as surgery or ESWL treatment (see Chapter 25).

What Are the Medications?

There are many different types of medications used to treat kidney stone disease.

1. *Alkaline potassium salts, including potassium citrate and potassium bicarbonate.*   The alkaline potassium salts are the most important medication used in the treatment of uric acid stones, and they play an important role in the management of calcium oxalate stone formers whose citrate (a natural inhibitor) excretion is low.

To prevent uric acid stone formation, alkaline potassium salts are used to raise the urinary pH to around 7.0. (See Chapter 3 on pH and Chapter 4 on uric acid stones.)

In addition, one treatment for managing calcium oxalate stone disease is to raise the urinary citrate. Potassium citrate compounds are used for this purpose. They are somewhat better than potassium bicarbonate compounds because they raise the urinary citrate level more.

Because potassium bicarbonate and potassium citrate are found normally in the body, these compounds might not even be called medicines. They are used simply to boost the levels of normal urinary components and are, therefore, a very benign form of treatment for most people.

They have very few side effects, but occasionally they cause stomach upset when first taken. Diluting them in lots of water or juice, or taking them over a period of an hour, can minimize this side effect if it occurs. One form of potassium citrate (Urocit K) comes as a wax-wrapped capsule that slowly releases the potassium citrate. Some people are unsettled by the pieces of wax they then pass in their stool. They are harmless.

Occasionally, alkaline potassium salts will produce diarrhea, particularly in people with *ileostomies*. In some instances, people who take potassium citrate or bicarbonate experience a spacey sensation for fifteen to twenty minutes. This feeling is caused by a momentary rise in the blood pH, which is similar to what happens if you hyperventilate. In both cases, blood pH rises, but for different reasons. If this effect occurs, I suggest taking the potassium citrate or bicarbonate over a period of an hour.

Alkaline potassium salts should not be taken by patients with significant kidney failure in whom too much potassium could cause a problem. Consult your doctor if you have any questions.

Some people decide that since some is good, more is better. Excess intake of an alkaline salt beyond the amount needed to raise your urinary pH to 7.0, or beyond what is prescribed for you, can make your blood pH stay in the alkaline range and make you feel terrible. Don't self-medicate or change doses without guidance.

2. *Alkaline sodium salts such as sodium bicarbonate.* This is baking soda. If you can tolerate alkaline potassium salts, they are better than alkaline sodium salts such as baking soda. However, some people cannot take as much of the potassium salts as they need without getting an upset stomach. In these cases, doctors frequently prescribe some of the alkaline salts as sodium bicarbonate or baking soda as long as the patient does not have high blood pressure or another reason to minimize sodium intake. You can use prescription sodium bicarbonate, but you can also measure out the baking soda you buy in a supermarket. Your physician can prescribe the amount of baking soda you should be taking.

With all the alkaline salts, the amount you need will vary with the amount of protein in your diet, as they are countering the acidic urine caused by protein metabolism. (See Chapter 8.)

3. *Thiazides.* The thiazide diuretics are used to reduce the urinary calcium in people who excrete excessive amounts of calcium. Thiazides include hydrochlorothiazide, trichlormethiazide, and the related chlorhalidone. These drugs were developed to lower blood pressure and to help people with edema (excess water retention) excrete excess salt. It was later found, in people who did not consume an excess of salt, that the thiazides would lower the urinary calcium. The last point is important: The thiazides will not lower urinary calcium unless dietary sodium intake is controlled.

We have discussed how an excess of salt causes an increase in the amount of calcium in the urine of all stone formers (see Chapter 8). In people who have a particularly high calcium excretion and in whom the doctor feels medication is needed to lower this urinary calcium, the thiazides have a role. However, control of salt intake is critical in such people.

The side effects of thiazides include potassium depletion. All people taking these diuretics must be sure that their diet contains enough potassium. Discuss this point with your doctor. Some people on thiazide diuretics will suffer from too low a blood pressure or from dehydration. In some circumstances, the thiazides can exacerbate a tendency toward diabetes and, rarely, cause attacks of gout.

For some chronic stone formers, the proper use of thiazides can markedly diminish a stone-forming tendency. Stone formers with *medullary sponge kidney* seem to do particularly well with thiazides, especially if they supplement potassium with potassium citrate.

4. *Allopurinol.* This medication reduces the body's production of uric acid. It lowers the blood uric acid level and also reduces the amount of uric acid excreted in the urine. It is the most useful medication in the prevention of gout caused by deposits of uric acid in joints and tissues (see Chapter 9). Its value in treating uric acid stones is less clear.

Allopurinol has some uncommon but potentially serious side effects, including a life-threatening skin rash and the suppression of white blood cells. Anyone who develops an unexplained rash while taking the drug should immediately stop the medication and contact a physician. For these reasons, the treatment of choice for uric acid stones is alkaline potassium salts and not Allopurinol. For a person with an unusually severe stone problem or a person who has gout, Allopurinol may be used along with the alkaline potassium salts.

Allopurinol is also sometimes used to treat calcium oxalate stone formers. A subgroup of these stone formers may have *hyperuricosuria,* or a high urate excretion in the urine. The urinary urate can act as a promoter of calcium oxalate crystals (see Chapter 8). Lowering the amount of urate excreted can make calcium oxalate stone formation less likely.

5. *Triamterene.* This is a weak diuretic that tends to raise the blood potassium. It has a mild tendency to lower urinary calcium. Unfortunately, triamterene itself is relatively insoluble in urine, and stones made of triamterene can form in people. While use of the drug in non–stone formers is common in the combination drug Dyazide and

is usually safe, it is not recommended for anyone who has made stones. Mixed calcium oxalate–triamterene stones have been reported.

6. *Amiloride.* This is a weak diuretic that was developed as a potassium-sparing diuretic. It is similar in action to triamterene and has a mild tendency to lower urinary calcium. Unlike triamterene, it is quite soluble in urine and does not make stones. In some circumstances, I have used it alone to reduce urinary calcium or in conjunction with a thiazide, which is more potent. The amiloride may counteract the tendency of the thiazide to lower the blood potassium yet still lower urinary calcium.

7. *Pyridoxine.* There is an uncommon inherited disorder called oxalosis where the body produces too much oxalate. (See Chapter 9.) One form of this hereditary disease improves somewhat with supplements of the vitamin B_6, or pyridoxine. A few adult stone formers with high oxalate excretions may decrease their oxalate excretion by taking pyridoxine supplements. But only a small fraction of stone formers will benefit from taking pyridoxine. Since high doses of the drug have been associated with neurological damage, this vitamin should not be taken indiscriminately. We may eventually find out that even small doses can be harmful. I recommend that the few stone formers with oxalate excretions over 45 milligrams every twenty-four hours who do not lower oxalate excretion enough with dietary changes ask their doctor about this vitamin. Sometimes its effects are dramatic. I do not recommend that stone formers take it without guidance from a physician and without demonstrating that they initially have very high levels of urinary oxalate.

8. *Magnesium oxide and other magnesium salts.* Magnesium is a weak inhibitor of the formation of calcium-containing kidney stones. In patients with severe diarrhea, magnesium supplements may be necessary for the health of the body. In these cases, magnesium oxide is the least likely to increase the diarrhea problem.

Some have advocated the use of magnesium to prevent stone disease in patients without severe diarrhea. No controlled trial has ever shown a benefit from such treatment, and at least one study has shown it to be ineffective. In people with diarrhea problems who have made stones, I sometimes give magnesium oxide. My goal is to restore normal magnesium levels in the body, not necessarily to use the magnesium as a stone preventative.

9. *Thiola and penicillamine.* These two compounds are used to treat *cystinuria*. They both reduce the total amount of cystine ex-

creted and make what is in the urine more soluble. Unfortunately, they have some important toxicities, including fevers, protein in the urine, and the destruction of white blood cells. Some people with cystinuria can take them without a problem and they provide dramatic control of the disease. These drugs should be given only under the direction of a physician experienced in their use.

10. *Acetohydroxamic acid.* I was involved in the development of this drug. It stops bacteria like *Proteus* from splitting the urea molecule and developing the changes in the urinary chemistry that predispose people to the formation of infection stones (see Chapter 4). The drug can inhibit the bacterial enzyme called urease, and clinical studies have proved it is quite effective in stopping the growth of infection stones and even in causing some of them to dissolve.

Unfortunately, this drug has some serious toxicities. It can cause blood clots within blood vessels and sometimes acute confusion.

11. *Antibiotics and urinary antiseptics.* If someone with retained kidney stones develops a simple bladder infection, the infection can climb into the kidneys where it is particularly dangerous (see Chapter 4). Women who have frequent urinary tract infections are often given urinary antiseptics like Hiprex or methenamine to minimize the likelihood of infections becoming established.

12. *Calcium citrate and other calcium preparations.* It is reasonable to ask why anyone would give calcium supplements to a patient who was making calcium kidney stones. However, the situation is complicated. (See Chapter 8, "The Calcium Controversy.") Calcium supplements often can help reduce the frequency of calcium oxalate stone disease in certain selected people with bowel problems.

Calcium supplements are also given to stone formers with a history of osteoporosis as well as stone disease. It is not unusual for the two problems to cluster in a family. My wife comes from this type of family and, when she complained that her nails broke too easily, she told me that her dermatologist had suggested that she take calcium supplements. She said to me, "Since you're the specialist, why don't you figure out a safe way for me to take calcium, not get another kidney stone and, more importantly, not end up with the bone problems my mother has." So we began a study of women who had previously made stones who were now past age forty and were worried about developing osteoporosis. We gave these women calcium citrate and followed their urinary chemistries very carefully. On the average, urinary calciums rose, but urinary citrates also rose and urinary oxalates fell somewhat. The net effect on urinary chemistry was no change in the stone-forming potential of the urine. Nothing in this study should be construed as saying it is safe for all women with stone disease to take calcium citrate. But there certainly may be some women whose stone history is distant in time and whose risk of osteoporosis is judged by the physician to be greater than the risk of stone disease. These women may benefit from taking calcium supplements. If you have made stones and are considering taking calcium supplements, you should discuss this question with your doctor.

13. *Phosphates.*   In some people, use of phosphate supplements may reduce the stone-forming potential of the urine; these supplements cause an increase in an inhibitor called pyrophosphate. However, since some stones contain phosphate, including *apatite* and *struvite* stones (see Chapter 4), phosphate supplements can be dangerous for certain people.

There is one situation where the use of oral phosphates is clearly indicated. In certain families there is a tendency for the blood phosphate level to be too low. People from these families frequently make calcium oxalate stones, and phosphate supplements are the mainstay of their therapy.

14. *Cellulose phosphate.*   Some stone formers absorb a greater fraction of the calcium in their intestine than other people. This is called *absorptive hypercalciuria*. In these hyperabsorbers, cellulose phosphate decreases the incidence of stone disease by binding to calcium in the intestine, making it unavailable for absorption. (See Chapter 9.) The trouble with this type of therapy is that it makes less calcium available for bone formation. Since many stone formers have less than normal bone densities to start with, and may come from families where there is osteoporosis, this type of therapy may have long-term consequences for the health of the skeleton.

15. *Aluminium hydroxide.*   This medication is occasionally used to treat patients with infection stones. The rationale for its use is that such stones contain large amounts of phosphorus. Aluminum hydroxide inhibits the absorption of phosphorus in the intestine and hence reduces the amount of phosphorus in the urine.

25

TECHNOLOGY

Old and New

*. . . these kidney stone operations are . . . sufficient to
deter any sufferer from undergoing an operation except
for the relief of a condition which is in itself worse than
death.*

—THE PEOPLE'S COMMON SENSE MEDICAL ADVISOR (1895)

Most kidney stones pass spontaneously. Unfortunately, some stones
become stuck and must be broken up before they will pass or are
surgically removed.

Procedures for "stones" are documented as far back as ancient
Mesopotamia. Cuneiform tablets have survived describing the pour-
ing of potions directly into the urethra/penis through a bronze tube.
"Cutting for the stone," or lithotomy ("lith" means stone, "otomy"
means incision), was practiced throughout the Middle Ages. This was
the province of barber-surgeons and usually involved entering the
bladder through the abdomen. By the eighteenth century, an English
surgeon approached the kidneys directly.

Since most of the early operations were performed without modern
hygiene or anesthesia—getting the patient drunk was the only means
of making the procedure slightly less painful—surviving the operation was, in itself, a measure of success.

Today, less than 10 percent of the surgery performed for stones
in the past is still done. Several advances have made it possible to rid
people of most stones that will not pass without resorting to open
surgery. The goal of these procedures is to break up the stone so that

185

it will pass by itself or to remove it with instruments inserted into the kidney through the ureter. (See Figure 1, page 11.) The following is a brief description of the current technology in the area.

Procedures

Urologists perform several different types of procedures to deal with stones that cannot pass spontaneously.

Extracorporeal Shock Wave Lithotripsy (ESWL)

Extracorporeal Shock Wave Lithotripsy ("Extra" means outside the body, "litho" means stone, "tripsy" means crushing) uses shock waves to reduce a stone to fragments that can then pass in the urine. Formerly known as the "The Bathtub" because people were immersed in a water-filled tub, the ESWL procedure is now done with the patient lying on a table. The lithotripter is focused so that the shock waves concentrate on the stone with little or no damage to nearby tissue.

Two low-level X-ray devices locate the stone, enabling the physician to position you properly and monitor you during the treatment to determine if the stone is breaking up. During the procedure, which lasts approximately one hour, you receive an anesthetic to numb the area receiving the shock waves.

If the procedure is successful, the stone is broken up and can be flushed out with fluids. Approximately 5 percent of the people who go through this procedure require secondary procedures to facilitate passage of the stone fragments.

Cystoscopy and Ureteroscopy

A physician can pass a visualizing *cystoscope* through the urethra into the bladder or use a *ureteroscope*, which is an extension of the cystoscope, through the ureter and up into the kidney. (See Figure 9.) These narrow tubes enable the physician to see inside the body using a special lens and fiber-optic lighting system. The entire urinary tract can be seen through the ureteroscope and accessed without making an incision. The physician can then thread laser wires through the scope into the kidney to break up the stones. Laser beams can pulverize a stone when the stone can be seen visually; they will not penetrate human tissue like a shock wave.

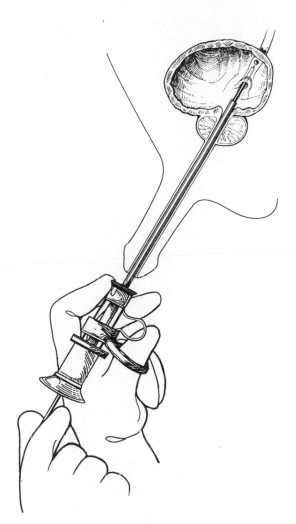

Figure 9.   Ureteroscopy
A surgeon enters the lower part of the ureter to remove a stone located there.

Percutaneous Nephrostomy Lithotripsy

For larger stones stuck in the kidney, it is possible to insert a *nephrostomy* tube through the skin into the kidney via a *percutaneous nephrostomy* ("percutaneous" means through the skin, a "nephrostomy" is a window into the kidney). An ultrasound or laser instrument is passed through the tube into the kidney and applied directly to the stone to break it up. (See Figure 10.) The physician can then pull out the fragments via the tube, which is about $^3/4$ of an inch or 2 centimeters in diameter.

In these procedures a stent or splinting catheter keeps the ureter open so the stone fragments can pass freely without blocking the ureter. New types of stents can keep the ureter open while uric acid stones, in particular, are dissolved.

Most procedures require, at most, an overnight hospital stay.

Surgery

There are still some stones that cannot be broken up by the ESWL or removed through any of the other procedures described earlier. In

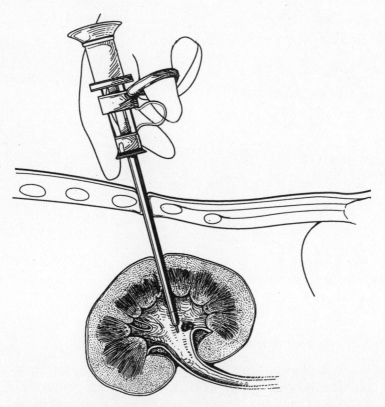

Figure 10.   Percutaneous Nephrostomy
The surgeon can use a tube placed through the skin and into the kidney to extract stones directly from the kidney.

these cases, the urologist must perform a *nephrolithotomy* ("Nephro" means kidney, "lith" means stone, "otomy" means incision).

Traditionally, to approach a stone in the kidney, the surgeon makes an incision in the flank, usually after removing part of a rib. If the stone is large, a cut is made into the kidney and a nephrolithotomy performed. If the stone is smaller than 1 centimeter or so, it is usually possible to cut only the pelvis of the kidney. This procedure is called a *pyelolithotomy* ("pyelo" means pelvis of the kidney). Finally, if the stone is stuck in the ureter, the surgeon usually approaches it with an incision to one side of the abdomen, just below the belly button. This procedure is called a *ureterolithotomy*. Like any open surgery, these procedures require several days of hospitalization and a postoperative recovery period.

Since this book is about *preventing* kidney stones, the purpose of this chapter is only to review some of the techniques so that you are familiar with the terminology. For a full explanation of all of the procedures, you should consult your urologist.

APPENDIX A
USEFUL TABLES

Table 1   Metric Conversion

Definition of Terms

gram	—	the basic measurement for weight, abbreviatcd as g
meter	—	the basic measurement for length, abbreviated as m
liter	—	the basic measurement for volume, abbreviated as l

Common Metric Prefixes

milli	—	a thousand times smaller, abbreviated as m
centi	—	a hundred times smaller, abbreviated as c
kilo	—	a thousand times larger, abbreviated as k

Common Conversion Factors

When you know:	And you want:	Multiply by:
quarts	liters	0.95
gallons	liters	3.79
ounces	grams	28.35
pounds	kilograms	0.45

**Table 2   Oxalate Content of Selected Foods
                (per ¹/₂-Cup Serving)**

Food Group	Use As Desired	Moderate Use
Beverages	Beer, bottled Carbonated cola (limit to 12 fl oz/day) Distilled alcohol Lemonade or limeade without peel Milk (whole, low-fat, or skim, and buttermilk) Wine (red, white, and rosé)	Coffee, brewed Coffee, instant (limit to 8 oz/day)
Breads and cereals	Breakfast cereals (cornflakes and oatmeal) Bread	Cornbread Spaghetti, canned in tomato sauce
Desserts	Ice Cream, ice milk, frozen yogurt, gelatins, sorbets, fruit ices (with allowed fruit fillings)	Sponge cake
Fats	Butter Margarine Mayonnaise Salad dressing Vegetable oils	

Fruits and fruit juices	Apple juice
	Avocado
	Banana
	Cherries, bing
	Grapefruit, fruit and juice
	Grapes, green
	Mangoes
	Melons:
	  Cantaloupe
	  Casaba
	  Honeydew
	  Watermelon
	Nectarines
	Peaches (Hiley)
	Plums (green or golden gage)
		Apples
		Apricots
		Black currants
		Oranges
		Peaches (Alberta, canned, Stokes)
		Pears
		Plums (Damson)
		Prunes (Italian)
		Pineapples
		Cranberry juice
		Grape juice
		Orange juice

Stop and Think	Avoid
Draft beer	Cocoa
	Tea
Grits (white corn)	Soybean crackers
Whole wheat bread	Wheat bran
Fruitcake	Chocolate
	Nuts:
	Almonds
	Cashews
	Peanuts and peanut oil
	Walnuts and walnut oil
Blackberries	Rhubarb
Blueberries	Strawberries
Currants, red	
Dewberries	
Fruit cocktail	
Grapes, purple	
Gooseberries	
Lemon, lime, and orange peels	
Tangerine	

(continued)

**Table 2   Oxalate Content of Selected Foods
(per $^1/_2$-Cup Serving)** *(continued)*

Food Group	Use As Desired	Moderate Use
Meat and meat substitutes	Beef Cheese Eggs Fish and shellfish Lamb Pork Poultry	Sardines Beef liver Beef kidneys
Potatoes and potato substitutes	White potatoes Rice Pasta	Spaghetti, canned in tomato sauce
Soups	Soups with allowed ingredients	Dehydrated chicken noodle soup
Vegetables	Avocado Brussels sprouts Cabbage, white Cauliflower, cooked Mushrooms Onions Peas, green, fresh or frozen Pumpkin Radishes	Asparagus Broccoli Carrots Corn Cucumber, peeled Endive Fennel Lettuce, iceberg Lima beans Parsnips Tomato and tomato juice Turnips
Miscellaneous	Coconut Jelly or preserves (from allowed fruit) Lemon, lime juice Sugar	

Stop and Think	Avoid
Baked beans canned in tomato sauce	Peanut butter
Tofu	
Sweet potatoes	
Gumbo	
Tomato soup	
Vegetable soup	
Beans (green, wax, or dried)	Beets:
Bok choy	Tops
Celery	Roots
Chive	Greens
Eggplant	Spinach
Escarole	Swiss chard
Leeks	
Mustard greens	
Okra	
Parsley	
Peppers (green)	
Rutabagas	
Summer squash	
Watercress	
Marmalade	

Table 3 Calcium

Recommended Daily Dietary Allowances of Calcium

Age Group	Daily Milligrams of Calcium
Adolescents and Young Adults:	
11 to 24 years	1200 to 1500
Men:	
25 to 64 years	1000
65 and over	1500
Women:	
25 to 64 years	1000
menopause to 64	
on estrogen replacement	1000
not taking estrogen	1500
65 and older	1500
pregnant and breastfeeding	1200 to 1500

Note: Stone formers should consult their doctors before altering their calcium intake.

Important Food Sources of Calcium

Best Choice per Serving Size	Worst Choice
Milk (1%, and skim), 1 cup	Chocolate milk
Ice milk (vanilla flavored), 1 cup	Ice cream (chocolate or strawberry flavored)
Yogurt (low-fat or fat-free), 1 cup, banana, lemon, vanilla flavoring	Whole-milk yogurt with the following fruit fillings: strawberry, raspberry, blueberry
Salmon, canned with bones, no added salt, 3 oz	Sardines in oil, canned with bones

Surprisingly, many nondairy foods rich in calcium are also high in oxalate and should be avoided.

Table 3   Calcium *(continued)*

Serving Sizes of Calcium- and Oxalate-Rich Foods

Food	Serving	Calcium (mg)	Oxalate Content	
			Moderate	High
Meat Alternative:				
Beans, cooked	1 cup	100		x
Sardines, canned with bones	3 oz	325	x	
Tofu processed with calcium sulfate	$^1/_2$ cup	130		x
Nuts:				
Almonds	1 ounce	70		x
Vegetables:				
Bok choy	$^1/_2$ cup	80		x
Collard Greens	$^1/_2$ cup	179		x
Kale	$^1/_2$ cup	90		x
Okra	$^1/_2$ cup	88		x
Spinach	$^1/_2$ cup	139		x

Source: J. A. T. Pennington, *Bowes & Church's Food Values of Portions Commonly Used*, 16th ed. (Philadelphia: J. B. Lippincott Co., 1994).

Table 4   Sodium

High-Sodium Foods to Avoid

Food Group	Restrictions
Beverages	Commercially softened water
Breads and cereals	Salted varieties, i.e., salt sticks, salted pretzels
Meat items	Bacon, chipped beef, corned beef
	Cold cuts, ham, hot dogs, and sausage
	Sardines, anchovies, marinated herring
	Smoked, cured, salted, or canned meat, fish, or poultry
Potato or substitute	Commercial casserole mixes, potato mixes with added salt, and stuffing
	Instant rice and pasta mixes
	Salted potato chips and snacks
Soups	Dehydrated soups
	Gumbo soups
	Regular canned soups
Vegetables	Pickled vegetables in brine
	Regular canned vegetables
	Sauerkraut
Miscellaneous	Celery salt, garlic salt, onion salt, and seasoned salt
	Kosher salt, rock salt, and sea salt
	Monosodium glutamate (MSG)
	Seasoning containing salt

Sodium Levels of Flavor Enhancers and Flavorings

	Serving Size	Sodium Content
High Sodium		
Catsup	1 tbsp (15 g)	178 mg
Garlic salt	1 tsp (5 g)	1300 mg
Mustard	1 tsp	65 mg
Salsa	3 tbsp	300 mg
Seasoned salt	1 tsp	1300 mg
Soy sauce	1/4 cup	3074 mg
Worcestershire sauce	1 tbsp	234 mg
Low Sodium		
Cooking wine	3.5 fl oz	5 mg
Garlic powder	1 tsp	1 mg
Lemon juice, fresh	1 tbsp	0 mg
Onion powder	1 tsp	1 mg

Table 5   Protein

Daily Protein Allowance Based on Healthy Weight

Weight Range in Pounds	Daily Grams of Protein (0.8 g/kg of body weight)	Daily Allowance of Cooked Meat, Poultry, Fish, and Eggs in ounces (7 g protein per oz)
95 to 114	35 to 42	5 to 6
115 to 134	42 to 49	6 to 7
135 to 154	49 to 56	7 to 8
155 to 174	56 to 63	8 to 9
175 to 194	63 to 70	9 to 10
195 to 214	70 to 77	10 to 11
215 to 234	77 to 84	11 to 12
235 to 255	84 to 91	12 to 13

Protein Grams in Commonly Consumed Foods

Item	Protein (g)	Serving Size (oz)
Hamburger on bun, 1 large	22.5	5
Skim milk, 1 cup	8.4	8
Whole milk, 1 cup	8.0	8
Fruit yogurt, low-fat, 1 container	8.0	6
Tuna salad, ¹/₂ cup	32.9	7
Shrimp, cooked, 15 large	17.8	3
Salmon, Atlantic, cooked, 1 piece	21.6	3
Ham quiche	13.0	4.3
Beef frankfurter, 2	10.8	3.2
Pastrami, beef	19.6	4
Chicken, light and dark meat, no skin	25.0	3.5
Top sirloin beef	30.4	3.5
Lamb, loin	30.0	3.5
Pork, loin	29.4	3.5
Liver, beef, pan fried	26.7	3.5
Veal, loin, braised	30.2	3.5

(continued)

Table 5 Protein *(continued)*

Fast Foods

Item	Protein (g)	Serving Size (oz)
Kentucky Fried Chicken		
Breast	27.5	4
Drumstick	13.1	2
Thigh	17.9	4
McDonald's		
Egg McMuffin	18.2	5
Pork Sausage	8.4	2
Quarter Pounder with Cheese	28.5	6
Filet-O-Fish	13.8	5
Chocolate Lowfat Milk Shake	11.6	11
Chef's Salad	20.5	10
French Fries, medium	4.4	3
Pizza Hut		
Pan Pizza, 2 slices		
Cheese	30.0	7
Pepperoni	29.0	8
Supreme	32.0	9
Super Supreme	33.0	9
Taco Bell		
Beef Burrito/Red Sauce	25.0	7
Tostado/Red Sauce	9.0	6
Taco Bell Grande	18.0	10
Taco Salad/Salsa	34.0	21

Table 6 The Reference Hamburger

Food	Serving Size	Protein (g)	Burger Equivalent
Fast-food hamburger	1	12.3	1
McDonald's Quarter Pounder	1	23.1	2
Frankfurters (8 per 1 lb pkg)	2	13.8	1
T-bone steak, broiled lean	3.5 oz	28.1	$2^1/_3$
Shrimp, breaded and fried, 11 large	3 oz	18.2	$1^1/_2$
Chicken pot pie	1 slice	23.4	2
Pizza Hut cheese pizza	2 slices	34	3
Lamb chop	3.5 oz	25.2	2
2-egg omelet with ham/cheese	1	17.1	$1^1/_2$
KFC fried chicken extra crispy 1 center breast	1	33	$2^2/_3$
Ham-and-cheese sandwich	1	20.7	$1^2/_3$
Burger King fish fillet	1	20.0	$1^2/_3$
Tuna salad submarine sandwich	9 oz	29.7	$2^1/_2$
Submarine sandwich	1	21.9	$1^3/_4$
Steak sandwich	1	30.3	$2^1/_2$
Taco, large	9.3 oz	31.8	$2^1/_2$
Spaghetti with meatballs	1 cup	18.6	$1^1/_2$
Lasagna, beef, Campbell's	10 oz entrée	27.4	$2^1/_4$
Roasted chicken with skin	$^1/_2$ breast	29.2	$2^1/_4$

Source: J. A. T. Pennington, *Bowes & Church's Food Values of Portions Commonly Used*, 16th ed. (Philadelphia: J. B. Lippincott Co., 1994).

Table 7   Purine Content of Foods

Foods grouped according to purine content are listed in the following table. The normal diet contains from 600 to 1000 milligrams of purines daily. A low-purine diet is restricted to approximately 100 to 150 milligrams.

High Purine Content (100 to 1000 mg of purine per 3 oz serving of food)

Anchovies	Mackerel
Bouillon	Meat extracts
Brains	Mincemeat
Broth	Mussels
Consommé	Partridge
Goose	Roe
Gravy	Sardines
Heart	Scallops
Herring	Sweetbread
Kidney	Yeast, baker's and brewer's
Liver	

Moderate Purine Content (9 to 100 mg of purine per 3 oz of food)

Meat and Fish	*Vegetables*
(Except those in the table above)	
Fish	Asparagus
Poultry	Beans, dried
Meat	Lentils
Shellfish	Mushrooms
	Peas, dried
	Spinach

Low Purine Content

Bread, white, and crackers	Egg	Pickles
Butter or margarine	Fats (in moderation)	Popcorn
Cake and cookies	Fruit	Puddings
Carbonated beverages	Gelatin desserts	Relishes
Cereal beverages	Herbs	Rennet desserts
Cereals and cereal products	Ice Cream	Salt
Cheese	Macaroni	Sugar and sweets
Chocolate	Milk	Tea
Coffee	Noodles	Vegetables (except
Condiments	Nuts	those in table above)
Cornbread	Oil	Vinegar
Cream (in moderation)	Olives	White sauce
Custard		

Source: M. V. and L. K. Mahan, *Food, Nutrition, and Diet Therapy*, 8th ed. (Philadelphia: W. B. Saunders Company, 1992) 696.

APPENDIX B
FOOD DIARIES

A well-documented food diary will uncover not only the nutritional composition of your diet but also other important information about your eating habits and patterns that can affect stone formation.

This exercise is meant to capture all foods, beverages, and supplements in your diet in the exact quantities they are consumed. Nothing must be omitted. Include water, medications, and vitamin and mineral supplements. Include all meals, snacks, and beverages consumed anytime of the day or night. It is also useful to record the time the meal or snack was consumed.

Do not change your present eating habits during the collection of the food record. That means listing the half of a glazed chocolate donut picked at during a coffee break, the french fries shared with a friend, or the midnight snack eaten in a sleepy stupor. Do not forget to record that seemingly innocent noncaloric pot of tea. Everything counts and everything must be entered in your diary.

It is best to record at least two consecutive weekdays and one weekend day (i.e., Sunday, Monday, and Tuesday or Thursday, Friday, and Saturday). If you can face it, a full week is even better. Although keeping a food record is time-consuming, the more days recorded and the more data collected, the better the overall picture will be. Once the analysis is complete, a unique pattern of drinking and eating will emerge.

Beware of underestimating the quantity of foods you consume. A portion that you may consider "average" or "medium" size is more likely to be large or extra large.

A dietary history may reveal an obvious "offender" or patterns of eating and lifestyle that occur during certain periods of time—family affairs, vacations, seasons—that are the key contributing factor to stone disease.

The major patterns of eating and lifestyle that we look for include the following:

• Living circumstances
• Travel (airline food and beverages you usually consume)

- Vacations and business trips (changes in habits that may contribute to stone formation)
- Exercise and sports engaged in and foods eaten during these activities
- Weight changes
- Drastic changes in dietary habits (i.e., weight-loss regimes)
- Major events in the recent past that may alter eating and drinking habits

The blank food diary that follows is designed to track your daily food intake and categorize the five areas of major concern to the stone former:

1. Protein intake based on your healthy weight (see Table 5). Convert 1 ounce of meat, fish, chicken, and eggs into 7 grams of protein
2 Oxalate-rich foods
3. High-sodium foods
4. Calcium (see Table 3)
5. Fluids

After recording *everything* consumed in a day, place an "x" in the oxalate and sodium columns where appropriate and tally the results at the bottom of the page. Protein, calcium, and fluids must be tallied by serving size. This record will help identify how many "offending" foods you ate, as well as how successful you were in consuming the necessary amounts of fluid and calcium. See the sample "Good Day/ Bad Day" diaries as a guide.

By carefully monitoring your daily food intake in this way, you will develop a greater awareness of your eating patterns and habits. This will help you target the areas of your diet that need improvement.

Blank Food Diary for Stone Formers

Time	Food and Portion Size	Protein (g)	Oxalate-Rich Food	High Sodium	Calcium Serving	Fluids (fl oz)

A Bad Day's Food Diary

Time	Food and Portion Size	Protein (g)	Oxalate-Rich Food	High Sodium	Calcium Serving	Fluids (fl oz)
8:30 A.M.	Scrambled eggs, 2 oz	14				
	Bacon, 3 slices			x		
	English muffin, 1					
	Butter, 1 tsp					
	Raspberry jam, 2 tsp		x			
	Tea, steeped 3 minutes, 12 fl oz		x			12
	Whole milk, 2 fl oz				$1/4$	2
	Sugar, 2 tsp					
11:00 A.M.	Tea, steeped 3 minutes, 12 fl oz		x			12
	Whole milk, 2 fl oz				$1/4$	2
	Sugar, 2 tsp					
	Chocolate covered donut, 3 oz		x			
1:30 P.M.	Fast-food cheeseburger, 4 oz	29			1	
	Hamburger bun, 2 oz					
	Slice of onion, 1 oz					
	Catsup, 1 tbsp			x		
	Pickle, 1 oz			x		
	Strawberry milkshake, 12 oz	11	x	x	$1^1/2$	12
4:00 P.M.	Chocolate bar with peanuts, 3 oz		x			
8:00 P.M.	Roasted chicken breast, 8 oz	56				
	Cranberry sauce, 3 oz		x			
	Mashed potatoes, $1/2$ cup					
	Butter on potatoes, 1 tsp					
	Creamed spinach, 8 oz		x			
	Dinner roll, 1 each					
	Butter, 1 tsp					
	Salted food for flavor, 1 tsp			x		
	White wine, 12 fl oz					12
	Rhubarb pie, 1 slice		x			
	Tea, 6 fl oz		x			6
	Whole milk, 2 fl oz				$1/4$	2
11:00 P.M.	Chocolate milk, 8 oz	8	x		1	8
	Chocolate chip walnut cookies, 4		x			
Totals		118	12	5	$4^1/4$	68

A Good Day's Food Diary

Time	Food and Portion Size	Protein (g)	Oxalate-Rich Food	High Sodium	Calcium Serving	Fluids (fl oz)
8:30 A.M.	Orange juice, 4 oz diluted with 2 oz extra water					6
	Oatmeal, 3/4 cup					
	Banana, 1/2					
	Skim milk, 8 oz	8			1	8
	Herbal tea, 8 oz					8
	Tap water, 12 fl oz					12
9:00 A.M.	Tap water, 12 fl oz					12
11:00 A.M.	Nonfat yogurt, vanilla, 6 oz	9			3/4	
	Mineral water, 12 fl oz					12
1:00 P.M.	Red wine, 6 fl oz					6
	Pasta, 1 cup					
	Chopped tomatoes, 1/2 cup					
	Porcini mushrooms, 1/2 cup					
	Olive oil, 2 tbsp					
	Grated Parmesan cheese, 2 oz	14			1/4	
	Garlic bread, 1 slice					
	Coffee, 6 fl oz					6
	Cream, 1 fl oz					1
	Italian ice, lemon flavored, 3 oz					3
	Mineral water, 12 fl oz					12
4:00 P.M.	Seltzer, 12 fl oz					12
	Green grapes, 1/2 cup					
7:30 P.M.	Ice water, 12 fl oz					12
	Mixed lettuce salad, 4 oz					
	Oil and vinegar dressing, 1 tbsp					
	Roast chicken, no skin, 3 oz	21				
	Mashed potato, 1/2 cup					
	Peas, 1/2 cup					
	Dinner roll, 1					
	Butter, 1 tsp					
	Vanilla ice milk, 1 cup	5			1	
	Herbal tea, 6 fl oz					6
9:30 P.M.	Cherry jello, 1 cup					8
Totals		57	0	0	3	124

GLOSSARY

absorptive hypercalciuria A condition in which the intestine absorbs abnormally high amounts of calcium from food, resulting in an excessive excretion of calcium.

acetaminophen A generic name for analgesics used for pain management, including brands such as Tylenol. *See* **analgesic**.

acidosis A systemic disorder occurring when the pH of the blood is low and the urine is chronically acid.

amino acids Component of all of the proteins in the body. Methionine causes calcium excretion to increase. Glycine is metabolized directly to oxalate. This is why excessive protein increases both calcium and oxalate excretion.

ammonium Produced by the kidney to "bond" with acid and flush it out of the system.

ammonium acid urate stone A rare type of stone found in patients with a bowel problem that causes the kidney to make an unusually large amount of ammonium. Patients who abuse laxatives form this type of stone.

analgesic Any of a group of over-the-counter pain medications. *See* **ibuprofen, acetaminophen, NSAID**.

apatite A form of calcium found in kidney stones. It is also the form of calcium found in bones.

bioavailability Whether food is found in a form readily absorbable by the intestines.

bladder Structure in the urinary system composed of muscle where urine is stored until it is excreted.

bowel disease Includes conditions such as chronic diarrhea and Crohn's disease (ileitis).

BPH Benign prostatic hypertrophy. BPH is enlargement of the prostate gland.

bulimia   An eating disorder characterized by stuffing followed by fasting or vomiting.

butazolidin   An **NSAID**.

calculi   Plural of calculus, Latin for stone or pebble.

calyceal diverticulum   A calyx that has been distorted by disease causing stagnation of urine, which makes stone formation more likely.

calyces   Structure in collecting system of the kidney where urine accumulates. (Singular is calyx.)

carbonate apatite   A form of apatite, a calcium mineral found in kidney stones and bones.

cardiac muscle   Muscle found in the heart.

catheterization   When a tube is inserted through the urethra into the bladder.

chlamydia   A venereal disease.

chronic diarrhea   Persistent or constant diarrhea.

citrate   The most important natural inhibitor of calcium oxalate stones.

colic   Spasm of the smooth muscle.

colitis   Inflammation of the colon—a section of the intestine.

creatinine   A product of muscle metabolism. Used to measure overall kidney function.

Crohn's disease   An inflammatory condition of the small intestine.

cystinuria   An uncommon genetic disorder that causes the kidneys to excrete too much of the amino acid cystine in the urine. Cystine can form stones.

cystoscopy   A procedure that inserts a visualizing instrument into the bladder via the urethra to examine the bladder.

detrussor muscle   Muscle in the bladder that expels urine.

dialysis   Procedure where blood is removed from the body and cleaned by a machine. This process is needed when the kidneys are damaged to the point where they can no longer support life.

diarrhea   Loose feces containing a large amount of fluid that is normally absorbed into the system.

digestive system   The digestive system breaks down and metabolizes the food and fluids consumed. It consists of the mouth, stomach, intestines, and rectum.

DNA (deoxyribonucleic acid)   The genetic machinery of cells. Parts of DNA called purines are metabolized to uric acid.

extracorporeal shock wave lithotrispsy (ESWL)   A procedure using focused shock waves to disintegrate stones.

gonorrhea   A venereal disease that can cause blockages in the urethra, leading to bladder stones.

gout   A joint disease caused by uric acid deposits.

hydroxyapatite   A form of calcium found in kidney stones and bones.

hypercalciuria   Too much calcium in the urine.

hyperoxaluria   Increased oxalate excretion in the urine caused by excessive absorption of dietary oxalate; the most common cause is intestinal disease, but an inborn metabolic abnormality, which is very rare, can also cause it.

hyperparathyroidism   Condition where the amount of parathyroid hormone (PTH), which regulates calcium metabolism in the body, is secreted at an inappropriately high rate. The calcium in the bloodstream stays too high and spills into the urine, causing stone formation.

hyperuricosuria   An increased urinary excretion of uric acid.

ibuprofen   Generic name for an NSAID such as Advil, Motrin IB, or Nuprin.

idiopathic uric acid lithiasis   Uric acid stone disease. This term is used when no specific systemic disorder is identified as causing the stones. There is usually a defect in renal handling of acid that leads to a persistently acid urine.

ileitis   Crohn's disease.

ileostomy   When the colon has been removed, the end of the small bowel, called the ileum, is placed on the skin. The opening on the skin is called an ileostomy.

inflammatory bowel disease   Any of a number of conditions such as colitis, Crohn's disease, or chronic diarrhea.

IVP   Intravenous pyelogram. An X ray of the kidneys taken after an iodine dye is injected into a vein.

jackstones   Calcium oxalate stones. So-called because their sharp crystalline spikes look like those seen on a child's toy jacks.

ketosis   An accumulation of certain chemicals during starvation, rapid weight loss, or carbohydrate-poor diets. Ketosis results in a highly acidic urine and is bad for the stone former.

KUB film   X ray of kidneys, ureter, and bladder looking for radio-paque stones.

lithotripsy   A noninvasive procedure where shock waves are focused on a stone to break it up. The fragments are then flushed out with fluids.

lithotripter   Machine that breaks kidney stones into fragments. *See* **lithotripsy**.

medullary sponge kidney (MSK)   A congenital condition in which the final ducts leading to the collecting system of the kidneys are unusually broad. This causes a slow flow of urine, and stones tend to form in the dilated ducts.

multiple sclerosis   A neurological condition that sometimes affects bladder function.

nephrolithotomy   Surgical procedure where an incision is made in the kidney and stones are removed.

nephrons   Each kidney has approximately one million of these microscopic structures that filter the blood entering the kidney and remove what is not needed by the body and return the substances that are needed. The nephrons coalesce into tubes that lead to the renal pelvis.

nephrostomy   Literally, a window into the kidney. Physicians use a nephrostomy tube to feed laser wires or instruments into the kidney without resorting to open surgery.

NSAID   Nonsteroidal, anti-inflammatory drug such as ibuprofen or naproxen. *See* **analgesic**.

osteoporosis   Weak bones due to loss of calcium.

oxalosis   An inherited disorder of metabolism seen in young children where huge amounts of calcium oxalate accumulate in the kidneys, causing renal failure. Some adults with high oxalate excretions probably have a milder form of this disease.

papillae   The projections of the kidney into the renal pelvis. These can be damaged by excessive use of NSAIDS.

parathyroid hormone (PTH)   Regulates the metabolism of calcium in the body. Excreted by the parathyroid gland in response to the amount of calcium in the bloodstream.

percutaneous nephrostomy   Procedure where a hole is made in the skin and a channel passed into the kidney enabling the urologist to remove a stone.

phosphate   A mineral found in kidney stones and bones.

potassium citrate   A medication used to reduce stone frequency.

primary hyperoxaluria   Another name for oxalosis. It is a rare genetic disorder found mainly in children where the patient generates too much oxalate. Consequently, the oxalate enters the blood vessels and causes them to calcify. When it spills into the urine it can cause calcification of the kidney and the formation of a large number of stones.

prostatitis   Inflammation of the prostate gland causing symptoms such as urgency to urinate, frequent need to urinate, and weakened stream.

Proteus   Bacteria commonly found in the urinary tract that can split the urea molecule and cause formation of struvite stones. This is the most dangerous type of urinary infection for the stone former.

purines   Adenine and guanine are purines. They are nucleic acids found in DNA (deoxyribonucleic acid) and RNA (ribonucleic acid) that metabolize to uric acid. DNA and RNA are part of the genetic and protein synthesis machinery of all cells. Therefore, any meat that has many cells (innards, for example), breaks down into uric acid.

pyelolithotomy Procedure where an incision is made during surgery in the pelvis of the kidney to remove a stone.

pyelonephritis Frequent episodes of kidney infections.

radiolucent A stone such as a uric acid stone is radiolucent because it does not cast a shadow on plain X-ray studies.

radiopaque Something that is visible on plain X rays. A stone with calcium is radiopaque.

reflux Condition where urine in the bladder goes back into the kidney pelvis. Usually a result of a bladder defect, reflux predisposes some people to infection and kidney stones.

renal arteries Main blood vessels that carry blood from the heart into the kidneys.

renal capsule Capsule surrounding the kidney. Pain fibers in the renal capsule give a sense of soreness in the flank.

renal colic Involuntary spasm of the smooth muscle lining the urinary tract. Colic is the main severe pain people experience when passing a kidney stone.

renal (or kidney) pelvis The final collecting point for urine in the kidney. From there it enters the ureter for elimination through the bladder.

renal tubular acidosis An inherited defect in the ability of the kidneys to excrete acid and lower the urinary pH to normal levels.

renal veins Blood vessels that carry blood away from the kidneys to other parts of the body.

resorptive hypercalciuria The increase in urinary calcium caused by a breakdown of bone in the skeleton due to a lack of use. Commonly seen in spinal cord injuries and others.

RNA (ribonucleic acid) Part of the genetic and protein synthesis machinery of cells. Parts of RNA called purines are metabolized to uric acid.

sepsis   Infection of the bloodstream.

skeletal muscle   The muscle found in arms, legs, chest, and so on that moves the body and controls voluntary motions.

smooth muscle   The muscle that moves things around your inner organs and blood vessels. It lines the uterus, bile ducts, blood vessels, intestines, and urinary tract.

spinal stenosis   Narrowing of the lower part of the spinal canal, which causes it to press on the cord. Bladder functions may be abnormal.

staghorn calculi   Struvite stones have a branching appearance like the antlers of a male deer. They are sometimes called staghorn calculi.

struvite stones   Infection stones.

trigone   A triangulur muscle structure at the head of the bladder that seals the ureters when you urinate so that urine will not reenter the kidneys. Dysfunction of the trigone causes reflux of urine from the bladder upstream to the kidneys and can contribute to urinary infection.

triple phosphate stones   Struvite, or infected, stones. So-called triple phosphate because of the elements—magnesium, ammonium, and calcium—found in these stones.

ureter   The funnel and tube that connect each kidney to the bladder.

ureterolithotomy   Procedure where an incision is made below the belly button into the ureter and a stone is removed.

ureteroscopy   Insertion of a visualizing instrument through the urethra and bladder into the ureter in order to remove a stone.

urethra   Structure through which urine is eliminated from the bladder. In the male, the urethra passes through the prostate gland and the penis.

vesicle irritability   Pain felt when a kidney stone reaches the tunnel of the ureter through the bladder wall. Vesicle is an adjective referring to the bladder.

BIBLIOGRAPHY

Books

Bauer, W. W., M.D. *Potions, Remedies, and Old Wives' Tales*. New York: Doubleday, 1969.

Jacob, Dorothy. *Cures and Curses*. New York: Taplinger, 1967.

Meyer, Clarence. *American Folk Medicine*. NAL/Plume, 1973.

Pierce, R. V., M.D. *The People's Common Sense Medical Advisor in Plain English*. Buffalo: World Dispensary Medical Association, 1895.

Robertson, W. G., et al. "A Risk Factor Model of Stone Formation: Application to the Study of Epidemiological Factors in the Genesis of Calcium Stones." In *Urolithiasis Clinical and Basic Research*, edited by L. H. Smith. New York: Plenum Presses, 1981, 303–307.

Rodman, John S. "Struvite Stones." In *Renal Stone Disease*, edited by C. Y. C. Pak. Boston: Martinus Nijhoff Publishing, 1987.

Rodman, John S., R. E. Sosa, and M. A. Lopez. Chap. 44 in *Kidney Stones, Medical and Surgical Management*, edited by F. L. Coe, et al. Philadelphia: Lippincott-Raven Publishers, 1996.

Rose, G. Alan. *Urinary Stones: Clinical and Laboratory Aspects*. Baltimore: University Park Press, 1982.

Ryall, Rosemary et al., ed. *Urinary Stone: Proceedings of the Second International Urinary Stone Conference, Singapore, 1983*. New York: Churchill Livingstone, 1984.

Smith, Donald R., M.D. *General Urology*. Los Altos, California: Lange Medical Publications, 1969.

Articles

Borgi, Loris et al. "Hot Occupation and Nephrolithiasis." *The Journal of Urology* 150:1757–1760 (December 1993).

Breslau, N. A. et al. "Relationship of Animal Protein-Rich Diet to Kidney Stone Formation and Calcium Metabolism." *Journal of Clinical Endocrinology and Metabolism* 66, no. 1:140–146.

Brinkley, L. et al. "Bioavailability of Oxalate in Foods." *Urology* 17, no. 6:534–538 (June 1981).

Geller, Markham J. and Simon L. Cohen. "Kidney and Urinary Tract Disease in Ancient Babylonia, with Translations of the Cuneiform Sources." *Kidney International* 47:1811–1815 (1995).

Goldfarb, Stanley, M.D. "Diet and Nephrolithiasis." *University of Pennsylvania School of Medicine Annual Review* 45:235–243 (1994).

Hall, Phillip M., M.D. "Calcium Stones: Calcium Restriction Not Warranted." *Cleveland Clinic Journal of Medicine* 62, no. 1:71–72, (January, February 1995).

Massey, L. K., H. Roman-Smith, R. A. L. Sutton. "Effect of Dietary Oxalate and Calcium on Urinary Oxalate and Risk of Formation of Calcium Oxalate Kidney Stones." *Journal of the American Dietetic Association* 93, no. 8:901–906 (August 1993).

Massey, L. K. and R. A. L. Sutton. "Modification of Dietary Oxalate and Calcium Reduces Urinary Oxalate in Hyperoxaluric Patients with Kidney Stones." *Journal of the American Dietetic Association* 93, no. 11:1305–1307 (November 1993.)

McKay, Donald W., et al. "Herbal Tea: An Alternative to Regular Tea for Those Who Form Calcium Oxalate Stones." *Journal of the American Dietetic Association* 95, no. 3:360–361 (March 1995).

Pak, Charles Y. C. et al. "Dietary Management of Idiopathic Calcium Urolithiasis." *The Journal of Urology* 131:850–852 (1984).

"Prevention and Treatment of Kidney Stones." *National Institute of Health Consensus Development Conference Statement* 7, no. 1 (March 30, 1988).

Rodman, John S. "Management of Uric Acid Calculi in the Elderly Patient." *Geriatric Nephrology and Urology* 1:129–137 (1991).

———. "Nutrition and Kidney Stone Disease." *Current Concept and Perspectives in Nutrition* 4, no. 1 (January 1985).

———. "Prophylaxis of Uric Acid Stones with Alternate Day Doses of Alkaline Potassium Salts." *The Journal of Urology* 145:97–99 (January 1991).

Rodman, John S., John J. Williams, and Charles M. Peterson. "Dissolution of Uric Acid Calculi." *The Journal of Urology* 131:1039–1044 (1984).

INDEX

ABOUT THE AUTHORS

John S. Rodman, M.D., is an internationally recognized expert and researcher on kidney stone disease. He is Associate Clinical Professor of Medicine at Cornell University School of Medicine in New York City and a member of the attending staffs at New York Hospital and Lenox Hill Hospital. He has published extensively in the professional journals and medical textbooks and has lectured worldwide on kidney stone formation and treatment.

Cynthia Seidman, M.S., R.D., is director of Dietary Services at The Rockefeller University Hospital in New York City. She coordinates the design and development of all research diets at Rockefeller and has published in a number of professional journals. She is cochair of the Research Committee of the National GCRC Research Dietitians Association and is a member of the American Dietetic Association.

Rory Jones, an award-winning writer and television producer, has done extensive work on health and medical topics. She has developed educational programs as well as interactive multimedia for both adults and children.